Healthy
at Home

Healthy at Home

Get Well and Stay Well Without Prescriptions

TIERAONA LOW DOG, M.D.

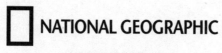

NATIONAL GEOGRAPHIC

WASHINGTON, D.C.

Published by the National Geographic Society
1145 17th Street N.W., Washington, D.C. 20036

Library of Congress Cataloging-in-Publication Data

Low Dog, Tieraona, author.
   Healthy at home : get well and stay well without prescriptions / Tieraona Low Dog, M.D.
      p. cm.
   Includes index.
ISBN 978-1-4262-1258-1 (hardback)
   1. Naturopathy. 2. Diet therapy. 3. Self-care, Health. I. Title.
   RZ440.L68 2014
   615.5'35--dc23

2013034581

The National Geographic Society is one of the world's largest nonprofit scientific and educational organizations. Its mission is to inspire people to care about the planet. Founded in 1888, the Society is member supported and offers a community for members to get closer to explorers, connect with other members, and help make a difference. The Society reaches more than 450 million people worldwide each month through *National Geographic* and other magazines; National Geographic Channel; television documentaries; music; radio; films; books; DVDs; maps; exhibitions; live events; school publishing programs; interactive media; and merchandise. National Geographic has funded more than 10,000 scientific research, conservation, and exploration projects and supports an education program promoting geographic literacy. For more information, visit www.nationalgeographic.com.

National Geographic Society
1145 17th Street N.W.
Washington, D.C. 20036-4688 U.S.A.

For information about special discounts for bulk purchases, please contact National Geographic Books Special Sales: ngspecsales@ngs.org

For rights or permissions inquiries, please contact National Geographic Books Subsidiary Rights: ngbookrights@ngs.org

Interior design: Katie Olsen

Printed in the United States of America

13/QGF-CML/1

For Mekoce and Kiara
and to all those who come after

Cherish the Earth
As you have cherished your own mother
Live your life in service to others
Give Glory to the Creator
Keep your heart close to Nature
Grow your roots deep
Be grateful for the Life you have been given
If you do these things,
Your Medicine will always be strong

Contents

Foreword

Studies of ancient peoples have shown that at least 50,000 years ago they understood the importance of plants in healing. In a recent archaeological study, Neanderthals were discovered to have residues of compounds found in chamomile and yarrow on their teeth. These are not food plants, so the investigators concluded that they were recognized by these people for their healing properties and used as medicines. The first known medical prescription, written on clay tablets by physicians in Sumer (modern-day Iraq) around 2400 B.C., describes the preparation of herbs as poultices and for internal remedies and offers guidance on other medical matters. This tradition of using plants to improve health and maintain wellness continues to the present day, with an estimated four billion people around the world relying on them for some aspect of their primary health care. And interest in this field continues to grow, along with an increase in laboratory and clinical studies evaluating the safety and efficacy of herbal medicines.

As an ethnobotanist I've spent most of my career learning about the uses of plants from indigenous cultures in remote parts of the world. This has been a journey that is now in its fourth decade, and I am fortunate to be able to continue these explorations. The pursuit of plants, along with knowledge about their use and conservation, has required long stays in areas that include the Amazon Valley, Central America, Asia, the Middle East, and most recently the small tropical islands of the Pacific known as Micronesia. In many of these places access to Western medicine is spotty at best, and often completely unavailable.

For example, the Micronesian islands are extremely remote and very small, and survival over many generations has meant developing a sustainable lifestyle in harmony with nature—after all, on an island of a few dozen or even a hundred square miles, if resources are depleted, there is nowhere else to go. At the same time, resilience is another requirement of the island lifestyle—people must weather storms, survive droughts, and deal with climate change and even an occasional epidemic of disease, while producing or importing the bulk of the things they need to live. In the arena of health care, many of these places are underserved, with limited facilities and access to modern pharmaceutical medicines. Thus, there still is great interest in using traditional, time-tested methods to treat common conditions and maintain wellness.

Over the past few years the teams of people with whom I've been privileged to work have produced primary health care manuals for the islands of Palau and Pohnpei in Micronesia, combining traditional plant-based healing techniques with contemporary medical practices. The idea is that by honoring and maintaining the health care approaches of the past, people can have a health care system that is sustainable as the elders who hold the knowledge pass on, and indeed, have a system that will withstand the transformations brought about by global change.

And it is that same spirit of self-sustainability and resilience amid the challenges of modern life that Tieraona Low Dog, M.D., provides the reader through this remarkably useful book.

A collection of lessons based on her experiences of growing, preparing, and using herbs—for patients, her family, and herself—this is an extraordinary resource for people interested in achieving a healthier lifestyle.

Healthy at Home: Get Well and Stay Well Without Prescriptions is a magnificent "how to" book for people who wish to make and use herbal medicines for the treatment of such common ailments as colds, coughs, insomnia, headaches, digestive disorders, and skin irritations, and in women's health. In this book Dr. Low Dog combines her herbal wisdom with her talents as a family physician, massage therapist, and midwife to teach, in easy-to-understand terms, how using herbs can reduce dependency on pharmaceuticals and over-the-counter medications, which in some cases, she points out, may not be as safe or effective as we think. At the same time Dr. Low Dog, an integrative physician, recognizes that there are times when people must turn toward allopathic medicine in search of a solution to their health issue. In this book she clearly points out the warning signs that let you know when more than self-care is necessary.

I've had the privilege of working with and knowing Dr. Low Dog for many years, since first meeting her at a course on the evidence-based use of herbs in clinical care that a group of us taught at the Columbia University College of Physicians and Surgeons. Her exceptional grasp of medical and herbal knowledge, as well as the skills and energy she brings to any project she is involved with, are impressive. And although she has been recognized with countless awards and honors over the years for her tireless efforts to improve the health care of those living in this country and abroad, she remains as modest and approachable as when I met her almost 20 years ago.

Healthy at Home: Get Well and Stay Well Without Prescriptions is a book that contains a lifetime of experiences with healing herbs and offers them to the reader—novice or expert—in a practical, engaging, easy-to-use, and fascinating format.

As she mentioned to me recently, "We are designed to be well, and I want to give people a renewed sense of awe in the amazing healing capacity of their bodies." This book delivers that awe, in the form of an effective and easy set of recipes designed to improve health and maintain maximum wellness. I learned many extraordinary lessons from this book and know that you will as well. I offer my thanks to Tieraona Low Dog, M.D., as I'm sure you will too after reading this book, for all that she is doing to change the way we think about health and wellness.

—MICHAEL J. BALICK, PH.D.
Vice President and Director, Institute of Economic Botany
The New York Botanical Garden
Bronx, New York

Introduction

My medicine road began when I was a child, and it has taken me from being an admirer of plants, to becoming an herbalist, a midwife, and eventually a physician. Some might say that the path I walked was unorthodox. It sure did have its share of turns and detours. But since the time I was very young, I've been fascinated by how the plants that grew in the gardens, forests, ditches, and streambeds could be used to help people heal their bodies. My grandma Jo said I came by plant medicine naturally. Her mother was skilled in using herbal medicines and was the person the doctor turned to when he needed the skills of a calm and wise woman to attend a birth or care for someone who was ill.

I opened up my first herb shop and herbal company shortly after moving to Las Cruces, New Mexico, in 1982. I spent roughly the next ten years making natural medicines and caring for those who sought my help. I watched in awe as children with recurrent ear infections and chronic eczema got stronger and healthier with simple dietary changes and gentle herbs. Many people who'd struggled with irritable bowel syndrome, indigestion, menstrual cramps, headaches, insomnia, back pain, arthritis, and depression got better. I felt good about the medicine I offered and my ability to be of service.

But the longer I practiced, the more I saw the limitations of natural medicine. I watched a woman die as untreated breast cancer ate its way into her chest. An elder woman slipped into a coma after trying to treat her severe hypothyroidism with seaweed, and a baby died of what was likely untreated meningitis. These experiences affected me deeply. I knew the time had come for me to pursue a medical education that would allow me to understand when, and how, to use the powerful tools of modern medicine.

And that's what I did. During my training at the University of New Mexico School of Medicine, my eyes were opened to the wondrous world of science. I was enamored with physiology. If I ever doubted that the body was designed for homeostasis and self-healing, those doubts had long vanished. I learned how to diagnose and treat patients with a wide range of disorders and diseases during my family practice residency. I witnessed first-hand the miracles of emergency medicine, surgery, and intensive care. I was, simply put, in awe of what modern medicine could offer. And I saw very clearly its limitations.

For all its magic in treating serious disease and trauma, for minor problems, it can often be like using a chain saw when a paring knife would do. These limitations are, however, exactly the strengths of natural medicine. Minor, self-limited conditions that are not life-threatening are highly amenable to this approach. However, in this modern age, we're increasingly at risk for losing the basic knowledge of how to maintain our health and the health of our families. We scurry off to the doctor's office for the most minor problems, becoming increasingly reliant on prescription drugs to help us sleep, suppress a cough, fight infection, squelch a rash, or soothe an upset stomach. Many people, particularly young parents, have virtually no confidence in their ability to distinguish between mild and minor conditions that can be cared for at home, and a serious or potentially dangerous illness that should to be managed in partnership with a qualified health care practitioner.

This confusion, in part, stems from the easy access to a wealth of health information and, unfortunately, easy access to much misinformation. It can be daunting to figure out what to believe. When I see advertisements for natural cancer cures or how to cure asthma using an ancient herb known only to shamans in the Amazonian jungle—I cringe. There are many things you can do to help your body fight off breast or colon cancer, but there aren't any natural cures at this time. Herbs have been used to treat asthma for thousands of years. Many reduce inflammation in the respiratory tract and dilate the bronchioles. However, the proliferation of products promising wonder cures from exotic, secret herbs known only to a select few are highly suspect.

As the fellowship director at the University of Arizona Center for Integrative Medicine, the nation's leading training program in integrative medicine, I have a strong commitment to evidence-based medicine. But we must look critically at the level of evidence required for each therapy and each condition. When a new drug is developed, it requires a robust set of studies because it is a substance that human beings have never experienced before. We need to understand how it works and the risks associated with its use. If the condition is one that could become dangerous if not appropriately treated, such as cancer or kidney failure, we must have good data supporting the drug's effectiveness.

However, when an herb has been safely and effectively used to treat minor conditions across many generations, I would argue that the same degree of modern research is not necessary. There are neither the resources nor the incentives to study all the natural medicines that are being used. If you're having trouble sleeping, trying chamomile or hops for a week, in my opinion, does not require the same degree of evidence necessary for a new prescription sleeping pill. Gargling with sage for a viral sore throat or taking ginger to settle an upset stomach should not need costly clinical trials before they are recommended.

As a physician who has used, researched, and recommended natural medicines for decades, I chose to write this book to help people gain confidence in treating minor problems at home using gentle and effective remedies. I have intentionally limited the conditions to those that do not generally require a visit to a health care practitioner for a diagnosis and/or treatment. I want to help you feel comfortable taking care of sore throats, colds and coughs, fevers, indigestion, diarrhea, cuts and wounds, rashes, and menstrual cramps at home. I want you to understand why using natural remedies that support your body's healing process is often better than using a more powerful intervention. Just as important, though, as a doctor, I want you to recognize when it is appropriate to seek medical attention.

I chose not to write a book that has an exhaustive list of every possible natural medicine that could ever be used to treat a given condition. There are plenty of those in the marketplace, and I've never found them particularly helpful. If there are 30 therapies for treating diarrhea, how am I supposed to discern which ones are the most effective? I find myself always wanting to ask the author, "Of these, which ONE would YOU use?" This is why I've only included those treatments that I've found most effective and safe in my practice.

When a treatment works 80 to 90 percent of the time without adverse effects, there is little need to experiment with every new supplement that comes along. Having said that, just because a remedy isn't listed in this book, it should not be inferred that it doesn't work. I've simply narrowed my recommendations to those that I have the most experience with, and confidence in.

With all of the quality issues surrounding herbal supplements in the marketplace, not to mention the cost, learning to make your own medicines at home has many advantages. You know exactly what is in your remedy and how and where it was made: your own kitchen with your own hands. Every section of this book provides specific instructions for how to make each remedy. And you can make it for a fraction of the cost of those sold in stores or online.

With this book as your guide, you'll be able to discern what you can care for at home and when it's time to seek medical attention. You'll learn to make medicines that are safe, gentle, and effective for just about any minor condition. These remedies can be used as first-line therapies, allowing you to avoid harsher, more potent drugs until they are absolutely necessary.

The title of this book says it all: *Healthy at Home.* Home itself is a sanctuary—a place to rest, to recover, and separate ourselves from the chaos of an often busy life. Home is the place where most medicine should start and finish. Physicians, like myself, can certainly be an important part of *healing,* but they should not be the primary source for your *well-being.*

My hope and prayer is that this book will empower you to take responsibility and control of your own health. To own the knowledge of healing and recognize the power of our body to heal is perhaps the most extraordinary gift that we have lost. We can each reclaim the self-healing powers inside of us, as we heal our loved ones and ourselves with all that nature has to offer.

◐ How to Use This Book

If you read this book from cover to cover, it will give you a new appreciation for just how well we have been designed for health and well-being. It's fascinating to step back and reflect on the many ingenious ways our body is able to defend itself from infection and disease. And more than a little disturbing to learn how our modern lifestyle and medicines can interrupt our body's natural forces.

Let me give you just a couple of examples: Many parts of our body are home to a staggeringly large number of microbes, with which we share a symbiotic relationship. They are vital to our health and our very survival. They assist us in extracting nutrients from our food, making certain vitamins, protecting us from infection, and maintaining the protective barrier function of our respiratory, digestive, and urinary tracts and skin.

Antibiotics are capable of destroying vast numbers of these beneficial microbes, sometimes taking months for their populations to recover, making us more vulnerable to future infections. The indiscriminate use of antibiotics in both humans and livestock has led to increasing numbers of bacteria that are resistant to their effects. Antibiotics are our modern warriors. We must use them wisely and only when absolutely necessary. If we continue on our current course, it will not be a question of "if" but only a question of "when" we will have a strain of bacteria that is resistant to all known treatments.

Many of the minor infections for which antibiotics are often prescribed can be easily and effectively treated using natural medicines that support the body's natural defense mechanisms without increasing bacterial resistance or destroying healthy microflora in the body. Throughout this book, I will help you discern what can be treated at home and when antibiotics might be necessary. And if you should need antibiotics, you'll learn how to minimize their negative impact.

Another common theme you will see in this book is the direct impact the nervous system has on our overall health. Whether dealing with eczema, recurring colds, diarrhea, or headaches— you can bet that stress makes it worse. More than that, we know that persistent stress can increase your risk for many diseases. Recognizing the true physiological consequences of chronic stress can be a real wake-up call for change. Although not a substitute for learning how to manage stress and make important lifestyle changes, plants have been used since ancient times to help calm, strengthen, and support our bodies and minds. Nervine relaxants, or herbs that relieve anxiety and promote a sense of calm, can be safely used without risk of habituation or side effects. Adaptogens, or herbs that help one adapt to environmental, physical, and mental stressors, may be more important now than at any other time in our history. I will show you how you can incorporate these into your life to improve your mood, energy, and immune response.

The first chapter is all about learning to make your own medicines. For those who grow or gather your herbs, information about harvesting and drying has been included. Resources for suppliers of superior quality bulk herbs have been provided for those wanting to purchase their herbs for medicine making. Always remember that your medicine can only be as good as the material you start with.

As you move through the chapter, step-by-step instructions will teach you how to make your own infusions, decoctions, tinctures, glycerites, medicinal honeys, oils, salves, and compresses. Although you might feel a little intimidated when making your first tincture—please be assured that I've taught thousands of people to make them at home in their own kitchen. If you can follow a simple recipe in a cookbook, I promise you can make your own herbal medicines.

After you've learned how to make your medicines, the bulk of the book is spent helping you learn to manage common health problems that arise in our everyday lives. Each chapter begins with an introductory section that briefly explores some of the key strategies the body uses to maintain its well-being. When these natural mechanisms are disrupted, illness can occur. Conversely, by supporting and strengthening these innate defenses, you can reduce the risk of getting sick. Then the specifics for conditions ranging from colds and headaches, to bug bites and heartburn, are discussed with detailed instructions for treatment provided. Just as important, at the end of each section, symptoms that warrant immediate medical attention are listed to help you discern when a situation has become too serious to care for at home. I've also included a section on when you should talk to your health care provider, for those symptoms that don't require a trip to the emergency room but do require follow-up. But remember to trust your intuition. If something inside says you should call the doctor or go to the urgent care—do it.

At the end of this book, you will find a chapter entitled "The Eighteen Essentials," where I have collated what I consider to be the most important herbal remedies to have on hand. Next you will find "Stocking the Pantry," which you can use as a guide for what you might want to keep in your home medicine cabinet. You will also find a list of resources for suppliers of herbs, seeds, and medicine-making items. And finally, the "Herbs for Today: A Modern Materia Medica" at the end of this book provides a brief overview of the uses and safety for the herbs discussed throughout the book. This is intended to be a quick reference. For more in-depth information, *National Geographic Complete Guide to Medicinal Herbs* is a good choice.

Chapter 1

Making Medicine at Home

I believe that making your own medicines is an empowering act. When I take or give my child a remedy that I have made with my own hands in my own kitchen, I feel deeply connected to my healing. The remedies I'll teach you to make come in many forms, from infusions to tinctures to salves. In this chapter, I will guide you through the basics so that you can gain confidence in your skills.

But before we get started, we should talk about the most important part of herbal medicine making, the herbs themselves. Your finished product will never be better than the starting material. What I mean by this is that the quality of the herb is critical: how it was grown, when it was harvested, and how it is dried and stored. My grandmother said that the manner in which the plant is gathered is just as important. One's frame of mind should be thoughtful and focused when harvesting medicine. Make your intention that these plants will be used with gratitude to help promote healing and well-being for you and your circle of family and friends.

Growing Your Own

I'm biased. I believe everyone should grow at least a few herbs at home. If you live in an apartment, you can have a couple of pots on your porch where you grow lemon balm, peppermint, sage, and thyme. These four herbs give you the ability to treat colds, coughs, sore throats, cold sores, nausea, diarrhea, upset stomach, gas, anxiety, insomnia, colic, bug bites, minor wounds, and even menopausal hot flashes!

Of course, if you have a yard, you can grow both veggies and medicinal herbs. There are few things in life more enjoyable than eating a tomato fresh or making cough syrup from thyme grown in your own garden. In "Resources" I've provided a small list of suppliers that I trust, where you can buy organic seeds and organic fresh plants to grow in your garden. These suppliers provide the correct genus and species, so you know that you are getting the right seeds. If purchasing from a local nursery, make sure you ask for the specific genus and species mentioned in this book. For instance, *Tagetes* is sold as marigold, but it is not *Calendula officinalis,* the pot marigold you want for your medicine.

If you're new to gardening, sign up for a class or two at your local nursery or botanical garden. I've learned so much from the horticulturists and gardeners who tend the plants. Most are more than willing to share what they know with someone eager to learn. Also, your county extension office can be a great resource for learning what plants will grow in your area, how to test your soil's pH, and so forth. In this modern Internet age, you can learn a great deal online, as well as from traditional gardening books. But there really isn't any substitute for spending a couple afternoons with someone who can *show* you the basics of gardening.

Remember, you're growing plants for food and medicine. Don't use harmful pesticides or fertilizers in your garden. Living on a ranch, I've been blessed with having all the chicken and horse manure I could ever need (or want) for fertilizer—make friends with a farmer, most are happy to share, if you're willing to haul.

Purchase or dig up some earthworms and put them in your beds. They'll work and turn the soil for you. Strategic placement of chicken wire and weed fabric can keep out gophers and squirrels, and cut down on weeding—all without the use of chemicals.

Gathering Your Herbs

When it comes time to harvest your herbs, investing in a good pair of gloves, long-sleeved shirt, and galoshes will come in very handy, trust me, for gathering things like raspberry leaves and nettles. You need a good pair of pruning shears and a basic pocketknife that will stay locked when open. If you've planted root medicines, a small shovel will make the job simpler. Then, of course, a basket to hold your delights!

The timing of your harvest is critically important. Leaves should be gathered in the morning after the dew has evaporated, when fully developed and before flowering. Leaves from biennial plants should be harvested in the second year, when the plant is not so heavily invested in developing its root system. Flowers should also be gathered in the morning after the dew has evaporated, just before they are fully open. Take fruits just before they are fully ripe, and harvest seeds when fully ripe. For those plants where all the aerial parts (leaves, stems, and flowers) are used medicinally (such as skullcap and California poppy), harvest the plant when it is in early flowering. Gather roots in the late fall after the aerial parts have died back. If the plant is a biennial, take the roots in the fall of the first year or early spring of the second. If a perennial, harvest the roots in the late fall when it is two to three years old. Barks can be harvested in the spring or fall, preferably from small or pruned branches. If harvesting the bark from the trunk of a tree, do not cut any more than a quarter of the trunk circumference to avoid harming it.

Certain plants should be used when they are fresh. Gather some peppermint leaves and make a cold infusion or harvest St. John's wort flowering tops to make a tincture. For those plants that you are going to dry, do so thoughtfully to preserve their color, potency, and essence. Make sure that you allow enough time to harvest, cut, and dry. Inspect your plants. Handle leaves and flowers delicately; bruising will turn them brown. Remove any bugs that might have come along for the ride. Leaves can be gently rinsed if dirty, but not flowers. Roots and stems can be scrubbed with a stiff brush. Don't let time elapse between the picking, cleaning, and drying.

Drying and Storing Your Bounty

There are a variety of ways to dry your plants. One of the simplest is to make a small bundle of your herbs (no thicker at the base than the opening of a beer bottle), tie with a rubber band, and hang on a string in a shady area that does not get direct sunlight but gets plenty of warm air. We hang ours in the "mudroom" where it always stays warm and there is no morning dew to rehydrate our drying plants. For roots and flowers, the easiest way to dry them is to put a couple of metal screens on cinder blocks and cover them with an old sheet or muslin cloth. These should be placed in a shady area where they won't get any direct sunlight but plenty of warm air above and below them. Do not cut your leaves or flowers. Whole dried herbs keep their potency much longer than those that are crushed or powdered.

The exception for this is large and/or fleshy roots, which should be cut transversely into small pieces, as this hastens the drying process and saves a lot of effort when it comes time to grind them for medicine making. Small roots can be left whole. Roots can be dried on drying racks, but I often dry all but the smallest roots in the oven at a temperature between 120 and 150 degrees. Leave the door ajar and turn every few hours. Cut open the root. Is there any moisture? Dry it longer. All plant parts should feel brittle and break when crushed or snap when bent. When completely dry, put them in an airtight container.

After your plants have been dried, inspect them again. Remove any damaged leaves, excess twigs, bugs, hair, and so forth. When finished, you're ready to store your herbs, preferably in airtight jars that you can store in a dark, cool place. Make sure you properly label the jar with the name of the herb and date of harvest. Leaves, flowers, herbs, and aromatic roots should be used within a year of harvest. Most other roots, seeds, and barks will stay good for two to three years, if stored in a cool, dark place.

Purchasing Medicinal Herbs

Gathering herbs from your garden is fun and wonderfully therapeutic, and you can also purchase fresh, organic culinary herbs such as thyme, sage, garlic, oregano, or ginger at many grocery stores. If you choose not to grow and harvest your own herbs, or want to make a recipe in this book from an herb that cannot be grown or located in your area, it's important to purchase from reputable suppliers. You may live in a town or city large enough to have an herb store, food cooperative, or natural foods grocery store where you can purchase herbs on-site. Are the herbs being sold certified organic or have they been ethically wildcrafted, meaning that the gatherer follows guidelines for not overharvesting, only gathering in the proper season, and not picking endangered species? Where are the herbs stored? Are they out of direct sunlight? Open the jar. Do the herbs look clean, colorful, and have a strong aroma? If you have any doubt, purchase elsewhere.

Compared with 20 years ago, it's easy to find companies on the Internet and order online or over the phone. In "Resources" I've provided the names of suppliers that sell certified organic/ethically wildcrafted herbs that you can purchase to make your home medicines. These are companies I trust. They have excellent quality control so you know you're getting the correct genus and species. Further, you can talk to people who are extremely knowledgeable about the herbs and their trade. The same rules for labeling

R̵X PRESCRIPTION FROM DR. LOW DOG
Gathering Your Own?

I gather many plants in the wild on my ranch; however, you should never harvest unfamiliar herbs. If you want to learn how to wildcraft, go and learn to identify the plants with someone with the expertise to teach you. Rangers, gardeners, botanists, and herbalists are great resources. Until you know what you are doing, stick with growing your herbs and/or purchasing from reputable suppliers.

---

and storing purchased herbs hold true—put the name and date of purchase on the label on your jar and store in a cool dark place.

OK, now that we've talked about the herbs themselves, let's get busy learning how to make the medicine!

◗ Herbal Teas: The Simplest Home Medicines

Medicinal teas, or tisanes, are the oldest method for making herbal remedies and one of the easiest ways to become familiar with various herbs and their benefits. From the delightfully delicious mints and chamomile, to the more potent echinacea and licorice, these preparations span the range from beverage to medicine. The difference relates to the choice of herb, the amount used, the length of time infused or simmered, and the frequency of dose.

Although I keep and use a good number of herbal tinctures (alcohol extractions) on hand in my medical practice and at home, water-based extracts remain one of my favorite ways to deliver and receive plant medicine. Teas can be nourishing and health promoting and are great alternatives to sodas and juice.

And they can be highly therapeutic. Drinking elderflower and mint tea is highly effective for easing a feverish cold, and hot chamomile tea is awesome for relaxation and sleep. My point is this: Don't underestimate the healing power of medicinal teas.

Before we get into the actual instructions for making these preparations, let's go over a few basics.

- *Fresh or dried*. Fresh herb teas are wonderful. I drink fresh lemon balm, mint, chamomile, and skullcap teas all throughout the summer. Many of the herbs mentioned in this book may be used fresh or dried. In a few cases, dried might be better. For example, the antinausea effects of ginger are more potent in the dried root/rhizome, while the laxative herb *Cascara sagrada* needs to be aged for several years to prevent severe intestinal cramping. In general, if the herbs are harvested at the correct time, carefully dried, and stored in an airtight container, such as a glass jar, leaves and flowers will keep their potency for a full year. Roots, stems, and bark will keep for several years.

- *Cut or powdered*. You'll want your herbs to be chopped into smallish pieces when preparing a tea. This allows a better extraction. You can also grind your herbs to a coarse powder right before making the tea; however, you'll need to strain it through a cloth to remove the powder or slowly pour the liquid off, leaving most of the powder behind.

- *Container*. When you are making herbal teas, the best vessels for preparation are ceramic, porcelain, or glass. Herbs, particularly those that are rich in tannins, can interact with metals, like cast iron or aluminum. If you have to use metal, choose stainless steel. For infusions, I recommend investing in a ceramic infusion mug that has a strainer that sits down in the water.

- *Water*. Soft and distilled water are best for making herbal teas. "Hard" water from a well or spring can form precipitates with compounds in your herbs.

- *Cook time.* The longer you steep or simmer an herb, the stronger and more bitter it will become, which can be upsetting to sensitive stomachs. In general, hard roots and stems need to be cooked longer than leaves and flowers, and plants that are highly aromatic should either be steeped for only about 5 minutes or prepared as a cold infusion (see the section titled "Infusions," below).
- *Preservation.* Teas do not contain preservatives, so they should be made fresh daily or refrigerated and used within three days.
- *Sweetening.* Adding honey, maple syrup, sugar, or stevia will not adversely affect the medicinal properties of herbal teas. However, if you are drinking a "bitter" tea for its stimulating effect on the digestive system, adding too much sweetener will reduce its benefit. Honey should not be used as a sweetener for any child under one year of age due to a rare but dangerous risk of infantile botulism. Maple syrup and sugar may be safely used in this age group.

Infusions: Healing Teas, Hot or Cold

Infusions are liquid preparations made by steeping fresh or dried herbs in hot or cold water. The liquid used is most commonly water, but could technically be wine, juice, milk, and so forth.

Infusions are ideal for soft, delicate plant parts, such as flowers, leaves, and nonwoody stems. Infusions are also recommended for roots like valerian and osha that are high in volatile or aromatic oils, which can be destroyed by prolonged heat.

Water extracts the medicinal properties from the herbs and brings out their flavor. Some herbs, however, are rather unpleasant tasting, and only the most hearty would drink them. I generally recommend saving the more acrid-tasting herbs for capsules, tinctures, honeys, or glycerites.

Directions for Basic Hot Infusion

To prepare: Bring water to a boil and let sit for 30 seconds and then pour over herbs that have been measured and placed in a container with a tight-fitting lid. Infusions are generally made using 1 to 3 teaspoons of the herb for every cup of water. Cover and steep for 5 to 10 minutes. The length of steeping depends upon the herb and the desired strength. Next, strain the infusion and drink slowly. Refrigerate any extra infusion and use within three days. Most infusions may be taken hot or cold.

Some of my favorite hot herbal infusions:

- *Chamomile flowers.* Beatrix Potter wove chamomile into her classic *The Tale of Peter Rabbit.* Known in Spanish as *manzanilla,* referring to its apple-like aroma, chamomile is one of my favorite teas for sleeplessness, anxiety, and upset stomach.
- *Lemon balm herb.* Also known as heart's delight and the gladdening herb during the Middle Ages, this delightful member of the mint family soothes and calms the nerves. Studies show that lemon balm alleviates anxiety and eases infant colic. It is safe for all ages, delicious hot or iced.
- *Nettle leaf.* This nourishing tea has long been used to ease inflammation. The German health authorities still endorse nettle leaves for easing arthritic complaints and soothing the urinary tract. Truly a "green" drink, nettle is suitable for the whole family. I generally drink mine iced and blended with mint.
- *Oatstraw.* Mildly sweet, oatstraw and the green tops of oats help ease anxiety and stress, a true tonic for the nerves. The herb is a "food" herb, very safe and can be consumed and enjoyed liberally by all ages.
- *Raspberry leaf.* Long considered a tonic for women, raspberry leaf is recommended by more than 60 percent of American and Australian midwives, according to surveys. It is widely used to reduce heavy menstrual bleeding and

to ease cramping. It contains a variety of vitamins and minerals and is nutritious for anyone. I mix it with other herbs such as mint and nettles, and drink it as iced tea.

Cold Infusions: Slow and Steady

Although most infusions involve steeping an herb in hot water, some herbs are best extracted in room-temperature water and left to sit for 1 to 8 hours. These include herbs that are highly aromatic such as peppermint or rich in mucilage like marshmallow. And it doesn't matter if it is a leaf or a root. The medicinal value of these plants can be compromised by excessive or prolonged exposure to heat.

Be aware that cold infusions run a small risk of bacteria or mold contamination—for two reasons. First, you're not subjecting the plant to the disinfecting effect of boiling or hot water. Second, herbs are generally not washed the way fruits and vegetables usually are. The risk, however, is a problem only for people whose immune system is compromised, for example, if they are undergoing cancer treatment, taking steroids, being treated with immune suppressants, or are young babies. In such cases, prepare the cold infusion; after straining, gently heat the tea for 5 minutes, but do not boil.

Directions for Basic Cold Infusion

To prepare: Place the herbs in a container with a tight-fitting lid and pour room-temperature filtered water over the herbs. Infusions are generally made using 1 to 3 teaspoons of herb for every cup of water. Let sit, covered, for 1 to 8 hours depending upon the herb and strength desired. Strain the infusion through a tea strainer. Use it immediately, or store it for up to 72 hours in the refrigerator.

Herbs made best with cold infusion:

- *Lavender flowers.* For occasional insomnia and restlessness, this herb can also be used topically for minor cuts and scrapes. Use 1 teaspoon per cup.

- *Marshmallow leaf and root.* A little slimy but that's because all those mucopolysaccharides in the plant are what coat, soothe, and protect the throat, esophagus, and stomach. Marshmallow is phenomenal for relieving occasional heartburn.
- *Peppermint leaf.* Much tastier as a cold infusion, peppermint can soothe a cough, ease a headache, settle an upset stomach, or be used as a compress to soothe a bug bite or strained muscle.
- *Slippery elm bark.* This herb can be used just like marshmallow. Use 1 teaspoon per cup. Add a pinch of cinnamon or maple syrup for a tasty drink.

R℞ PRESCRIPTION FROM DR. LOW DOG
Herbal Ice Cubes

I make a cold peppermint infusion by steeping 4 tea bags or 4 teaspoons of dried peppermint or a small handful of fresh peppermint leaves in 4 cups room-temperature water for 2 to 4 hours. Then I strain the herbs out and pour the liquid into my ice cube trays. If I have any fruit handy, I'll put a raspberry or sliced strawberry in each ice cube slot to enhance the appearance. After these are frozen, I'll empty them into a freezer bag for future use. Peppermint ice cubes are great for easing gas and indigestion, are lovely added to a glass of water, can be used to make an herbal compress for headaches or sore muscles, or can even be rubbed on an insect bite to take out the itch and sting.

I suggest keeping chamomile ice cubes on hand, especially if you have kids. They can be made into ice chips to ease nausea and diarrhea or put into smoothies to soothe a stressed-out first grader.

Decoctions: Drawing Out the Healing Power

"Decoction" is derived from the Latin *decoquere,* which means "to boil." Decoctions are the most popular method for preparing herbal medicines worldwide, particularly in traditional Chinese medicine (TCM). A decoction is a liquid preparation that is made by simmering fresh or dried herbs in water, or another fluid.

Decoctions are suitable for hard, tough plant parts, including barks, woody stems, most roots, and some berries. Prolonged heat is especially necessary to rehydrate dried roots and barks, which allows for maximum extraction of water-soluble parts of the plant. Roots and seeds that are highly aromatic, like osha or valerian, or that contain mucilage, such as marshmallow root and slippery elm bark, should not be decocted. The excessive heat will dramatically lessen the medicinal benefits.

Always begin your decoction with cold water. Immersing woody herbs immediately in hot water can congeal the albumin within the cell wall, impairing release of the herb's constituents into the water.

Directions for Basic Herbal Decoction

To prepare: Medicinal-strength decoctions are generally made by placing 1 ounce (a small handful) of finely chopped or newly powdered herb in 32 ounces of room-temperature water and letting sit for 60 minutes. Then bring the mixture to a boil, simmer covered for 10 to 30 minutes, and then strain. Decoctions should be used immediately or stored up to 72 hours in the refrigerator. Some of my favorite herbs for decoctions:

- *Burdock root.* Known as "gobo" in Japan, burdock is eaten as a root vegetable in many Asian countries. It strengthens the liver's natural detoxification processes and has been used for centuries to improve skin and gut health. Rich in the prebiotic inulin, burdock makes a great soup base. Drink or eat as desired.

- *Dandelion root.* Historically, the leaves were cooked and eaten as a vegetable and the roots dried and roasted as a coffee substitute (though no coffee lover would find it a great alternative). Rich in the prebiotic inulin, dandelion root has mild stool-softening effects and reliable liver-protecting properties. Drink 1 to 3 cups a day, as desired.

- *Echinacea root.* Although most people like the tincture, the tea is highly effective for relieving sore throats and helping the body fight off a cold or upper respiratory infection if taken at the onset of getting sick.

- *Ginger rhizome/root.* Few things are more delicious than fresh ginger tea. It's great alone or with honey and lemon for relieving symptoms of a cold, soothing a sore throat, or warming up your fingers and toes on a cold night. Drink 1 to 3 cups a day.

- *Licorice root.* This herb has been highly prized for both its flavor and medicinal properties since ancient times. It thins mucus, making it easier to expectorate, soothes the throat and stomach, and has potent antiviral and anti-inflammatory activity. It is best taken in doses of ¼ cup 3 to 4 times a day for only a few days, because prolonged use can elevate blood pressure.

◗ Herbal Compresses: Soothing From the Outside In

Check the pharmacy shelves: There's certainly no shortage of over-the-counter (OTC) medicines to treat headaches, stuffy noses, or muscle aches. Unfortunately, many of these drugs may impede the body's natural ability to heal itself and can have side effects. Acetaminophen, an OTC painkiller, is now the leading cause of acute liver failure in the United States. High doses and/or prolonged use of ibuprofen, naproxen, and aspirin can damage kidneys and cause the stomach to bleed. Nasal decongestant sprays can cause rebound, making your nasal passages swell and your stuffy nose even worse. Natural remedies, on the other hand, tend to have milder effects and fewer side effects, and support your body's recovery process.

One of my favorite treatments is the compress, also known as a fomentation, which is made by soaking a cloth in herbal liquid and applying topically to the skin. The liquid can be hot or cold, depending upon what you're treating. Cold compresses are used to soothe a headache, relieve the pain and swelling of a strain or sprain, or to reducing swelling and bleeding from a wound. Hot compresses are used to relieve pain when there isn't significant swelling or inflammation. Moist heat penetrates more effectively than dry, making hot compresses very helpful for chronic back pain or muscle tightness.

Directions for Basic Herbal Compress

Begin with 2 tablespoons fresh herb or 1 tablespoon dried herb and prepare an infusion or decoction, depending upon the herb, as directed in the section above on herbal teas. Strain. Add a couple of ice cubes if the injury came on suddenly and you want to reduce pain, swelling, and inflammation. Soak a soft cotton or flannel cloth in the liquid, wring, and apply to the injury. If the injury is more than 24 to 48 hours old, apply the compress and then cover with a hot water bottle or heating pad set on low temperature.

You can also use essential oils or tinctures. Begin with 15 to 20 drops essential oil or 1 teaspoon herbal tincture. Simply add to water and proceed as described above.

Compresses are typically applied for 20 minutes and then removed for 10 to 20 minutes. The cloth is dipped into the liquid again and reapplied for an additional 20 minutes. Repeat this procedure 2 to 3 times a day, or as needed.

Some of my favorite herbal compresses are:

- *Peppermint compress.* When I was a massage therapist, I often applied hot peppermint compresses to relax tense muscles in the neck and shoulders of my clients. Cold peppermint compresses for easing headache or sinus congestion are one of the basic preparations I teach the clinicians who come through the fellowship program at the Arizona Center for Integrative Medicine.

- *Arnica compress.* Arnica became one of my closest herbal allies when I was taking tae kwon do (martial arts) classes. Occasionally during sparring, I'd bang my shin or forearm, and right after class, I'd head for my kitchen, put some arnica tincture in a bowl of water, throw in a few ice cubes, and apply the compress to my exquisitely painful, bruised tissue. After a couple hours, the swelling would subside, and the reddish blue hue of my skin would start to fade. The relief I felt was nothing short of magical. Note: Do not use arnica topically for more than 10 to 14 days. Discontinue use if your skin develops a sensitivity or rash. Do not use arnica on open wounds.

◉ Herbal Honeys: How Sweet It Is

It took me a while to figure out that medicine doesn't have to always taste terrible, and it doesn't have to be a battle every time you want to give your five-year-old something to reduce a fever or ease a cough. Now I know that Mary Poppins had it right: A spoonful of sugar, or honey, can definitely help the medicine go down—which is why I keep a variety of medicinal honeys in my pantry and readily dispense them to patients and family alike.

Honey is prized as much for its medicinal properties as for its sweet taste. It has long been considered a healing agent. It is as effective as any over-the-counter cough remedy, and relieves sore throats. It is an amazing wound healer, keeping abrasions and burns moist, preventing infection, stimulating tissue regeneration, and reducing scarring.

The delectable nectars in this section blur the line between food and medicine. Lavender honey drizzled over cheese is delicious but can also soothe and relax you. Thyme honey over carrots will have the most finicky child asking for more and is highly effective for easing coughs and congestion.

When making honeys that I am going to use in cooking, I often use local clover honey as a base because of its mild flavor. Otherwise, I love the dark-colored honeys for medicine. I recommend "local" because, like wine and produce, honey carries the unique flavor of the land where the particular bees live and of the flowers that grow there. Use only raw honey. Pasteurized honey sold at most grocery stores has been heated, destroying the enzyme glucose oxidase, which accounts for the honey's powerful effects. Contrary to what you might have heard, local honey isn't usually that helpful for most people with seasonal allergies. The pollen from many nonflowering trees, grasses, and weeds are what cause that old familiar sneezing and stuffy nose for most of us, and these do not constitute the majority of pollen gathered by bees. (In other words, you don't find local ragweed or pine honey!)

Directions for Basic Herb-Infused Honey

Begin with ¼ to ½ cup fresh chopped herb (or half this amount if you are using dried) and 1 to 1¼ cups (8 to 10 ounces) honey.

Pour the honey into a saucepan and gently heat. Add the herbs and stir. If you don't like to fuss with sticky herbs, you can always put the herbs in a little cloth bag or tea ball to keep them contained and easier to strain.

Pour your gently heated herbal honey into a clean jar, cover with a lid, and let sit in a warm place (windowsill) for 2 to 3 weeks. Take off the lid and put the jar into a saucepan with water. Gently heat the jar until the honey has become liquid. Pour through a fine-mesh strainer to remove the herbs. Then pour the honey into a clean jar, label, and store in a cool dark cabinet. Your herbal honey will keep for at least one year.

Some of my favorite herbal honeys are:

- *Sage honey.* I grow sage year-round to use for both cooking and medicine. Sage is best known for its talents as a spice for chicken and turkey, but it is also an amazing medicinal herb. For a sore throat, bring 1 cup water to a near boil, pour over 1 teaspoon sage honey, and add the juice of half a lemon. Drink slowly and enjoy. Repeat 3 to 4 times a day, as needed. You'll feel better in no time! Of course, you can also take the honey straight off the spoon. It's delicious! Sage honey makes a powerful and effective wound dressing. Once the wound has been thoroughly cleaned, you can apply this honey to a gauze dressing and cover. (See Chapter 6 for more details.)

- *Lavender honey.* Few elixirs are more lovely and luscious than lavender honey. I use ¼ cup lavender flowers when making mine, as lavender, while lovely, can be strong. I love a little mixed with a couple drops of pure vanilla extract and fresh berries in organic plain yogurt! Your guests and family alike will love lavender honey drizzled on slices of Spanish Manchego cheese. Or take ¼ cup of your honey and mix with 1 cup sea salt or sugar and 1 cup olive oil to make a lavender/honey body scrub that is nothing short of divine.

- *Thyme honey.* Here's an herbal powerhouse for fighting off upper respiratory infections. Just add 1 teaspoon thyme honey to a cup of hot water with lemon. For nutrition, it's a favorite around my house on cooked carrots or mixed with goat cheese and served with whole grain crackers or warm bread.

WARNING: Honey and corn syrup should not be given to babies under the age of 12 months due to the risk of botulism. Although infantile botulism is exceedingly rare, don't chance it. Use maple syrup instead. According to the Centers for Disease Control, the risk of botulism from maple syrup is highly unlikely and is a much better choice for young infants.

▶ Herbal Tinctures: The Essence of Home Healing

Once the ancients learned to distill alcohol, it wasn't long until they figured out it could be used to effectively extract and preserve medicinal herbs. Tincture is the proper name for an herbal preparation produced using a mixture of alcohol and water as the solvent, or menstruum (the more precise term for a solvent used to extract compounds from a plant). They are still used in modern medicine and are also widely available at health food stores and herb shops. Tinctures are a highly convenient way of taking herbs, and the combination of alcohol and water can dissolve and extract virtually all constituents in the plant. Alcohol is also a great preservative, giving your herbal medicine a long shelf life, often more than 10 years if stored in a cool, dark place.

There are a couple of disadvantages to using tinctures. The first is cost, particularly in the United States where tincture prices are approximately 2 to 3 times more than anywhere else in the world. But by learning how to make your own tinctures, you can make them for a fraction of what you'd pay at the store. The second is that some people don't want, or are unable, to consume alcohol. This is easily remedied by using glycerin instead of alcohol as your solvent (see "Herbal Glycerites," page 45).

Tinctures are an important part of any home medicine chest, being invaluable for first aid and acute situations. So let's dive in! To get started, let's go over some terminology and basics.

Making Tinctures

Maceration and percolation are the two primary methods for making tinctures; however, I will only focus on the maceration method because it works well and doesn't require any special or expensive equipment. Maceration is the addition of a known quantity and strength of menstruum to a known weight of herb. The herb is cut or ground to a coarse ground powder and then mixed with the menstruum. The mixture is then allowed to sit for approximately 2 weeks. This prolonged contact between the alcohol/water mixture and the herb makes the extraction almost complete, allowing a highly efficient use of the herb, cutting down on the waste of our most valuable resource, the herbs themselves. It also means that relatively small doses of tincture have a similar activity to a large cup of infusion. After 2 weeks, the herbs are pressed, and the liquid filtered and bottled. The "spent" herb, known as the "marc," may then be used as an excellent compost.

The menstruum, or solvent, that is generally used to make a tincture is alcohol and water, though it can also be vinegar, honey, or glycerin. (See glycerin tinctures, also known as glycerites, pages 45–49, and medicinal honeys, pages 35–38.) Here we will focus on alcohol.

To be a tincture, the menstruum ratio must be greater than 1 —meaning that the volume of menstruum exceeds the weight of herb used. For example, a 1:5 tincture tells us that for every kilogram (1,000 grams) of herb, 5 liters of menstruum has been used (5,000 milliliters). That means 5 milliliters of finished tincture provides one gram of herb. For a 1:3 tincture, 3 milliliters of finished tincture provides 1 gram of herb. So, the lower the ratio, the more concentrated the tincture. Although I do not include any toxic plants in this book, by convention it is agreed that these are all made using a ratio of 1:10, meaning that 10 milliliters of finished tincture provides 1 gram of herb—this helps to reduce the risk of overdose and harm. The vast majority of tinctures in this book will have a ratio of 1:5.

Tincture Ingredients

Alcohol is a superior solvent and preservative, which makes it an excellent choice as a menstruum. The proportion of alcohol used in tinctures ranges from 25 percent to 90 percent, depending primarily on the active constituents we want to extract from the plant. Grain alcohol is 190 proof, which means it is 95 percent alcohol and 5 percent water. (Divide the proof by 2 to get the percentage of alcohol.) For ease and simplicity, just consider it 100 percent alcohol when making your extract—trust me, the math is easier and it won't affect your home remedy. Grain alcohol is versatile because you can use it to make a tincture containing 25 percent alcohol or one that is 90 percent alcohol, simply by how much you dilute it with water. Vodka is another excellent menstruum because it is available as 80 and 100 proof, meaning it is 40 percent alcohol and 60 percent water, and 50 percent alcohol and water, respectively. I also use brandy (80 proof) as I prefer the taste.

Tinctures can be made from either fresh or dried plant material, and instructions are given below for both. There are lots of

R
X PRESCRIPTION FROM DR. LOW DOG

Herb Vinegars

I am a huge fan of organic, raw apple cider vinegar for food and medicine. It is inexpensive, highly nutritious, pleasant tasting, and can be enjoyed by anyone. There are a few herbs that I always put up in vinegar including sage, cayenne, ginger, oregano, and thyme. I generally wilt my fresh herbs for a few hours or overnight to remove some of the water in the plant; I've found my vinegars keep better this way. Grind your freshly dried herb into a coarse powder, put in a jar, cover with organic apple cider vinegar (or wine vinegar, but never white vinegar), and let steep for 14 days. Then strain and bottle. This will keep for a minimum of one year.

opinions out there about which is better but I have to say that after 30 years of making both and giving them to patients, there are only a handful in which I've really noticed a difference. The main thing you have to keep in mind is that your finished tincture will only be as good as your starting material!

The tinctures I like to make primarily from fresh herbs include:

- Calendula flowers *(Calendula officinalis)*
- California poppy flowering herb *(Eschscholzia californica)*
- Corn silk *(Zea mays)*
- Dandelion root *(Taraxacum officinale)*
- Ginger rhizome *(Zingiber officinale)*
- Milky oat seed *(Avena sativa)*
- Nettle *(Urtica dioica)*
- Skullcap *(Scutellaria lateriflora)*
- St. John's wort *(Hypericum perforatum)*
- Turmeric root *(Curcuma longa)*

Tips Before Making Tinctures

The best vessels for making tinctures are widemouthed glass canning jars that have screw-down airtight lids that won't rust when they come into contact with alcohol, vinegar, or glycerin.

Tinctures being made with the maceration method must be agitated or shaken daily to keep the extraction process active. When using the maceration method, you must keep all the herbal material in contact with the menstruum. This means you'll want to regularly shake the tincture on a daily basis.

You need to let your tincture sit for a minimum of 14 days to get maximum extraction. It won't hurt to let them steep longer. When I'm busy, I'll just keep shaking them on the kitchen counter until I have some free time to press, filter, and bottle.

Tincture presses are available for purchase on the Internet for serious home medicine makers. Apple cider and wine presses can also be used. For most folks, though, some elbow grease along with cheesecloth/muslin, a strainer, and a bowl will suffice. Just layer a strainer with cloth over a bowl and pour all the contents from your jar into it. Let it sit for about 5 minutes and then gather up the cloth and squeeze repeatedly to get as much liquid out as possible. Then pour your liquid into a dark amber bottle and compost the marc, or spent herbs in your cloth.

Once you have pressed and bottled your herbs, make sure you label the bottle accurately and carefully with the herb name, date of tincture, and menstruum ratio (1:3, 1:5, and so on). Then store in a dark, cool cupboard. If using alcohol/water mixtures and stored properly, your tincture will remain good for many years. I've had some for 10 years that were almost as good as the day I made them. Vinegar tinctures keep for about 1 year, glycerin tinctures for 1 to 2 years.

Directions for Basic Fresh Herb Tincture

Some herbs are best tinctured when they are fresh, as some of their medicinal benefits are lost during the drying process. When making a tincture from fresh plant, you have to take into consideration the amount of water contained within the plant and adjust your specification accordingly. One kilogram (1,000 grams) fresh plant contains approximately 750 milliliters of water. This means that you must adjust the percentage of alcohol within your menstruum to obtain the correct finished solvency.

Here are the steps for preparing a fresh herb tincture:

1. Gently rinse off dirt from the leaves and flowers, and scrub roots. Weigh the herb on your scale, then finely chop it with a knife and put it in the blender.
2. If your menstruum ratio is 1:5 and you have 100 grams of fresh herb, you will then need 500 milliliters of menstruum (100 x 5 = 500 milliliters). For most plants, 50 percent alcohol will extract the medicinal compounds into solution. So you would need 250 milliliters of grain

alcohol plus 250 milliliters of water. Freshly harvested herbs contain about 75 percent of their weight in water, so your 100 grams of herb will be contributing 75 milliliters of water. Subtract 75 milliliters from the 250 milliliters and this means you will be adding 175 milliliters of water to your grain alcohol. This will result in a 1:5 extract containing 50 percent alcohol.

3. Turn on the blender and mix well. If you don't have a blender, you can always put the fresh herb and alcohol into your jar and then mix well with a wooden spoon. Make sure that the alcohol completely covers the herb.

4. Pour the liquid into your canning jar (make sure it is of sufficient size). Leave an inch or two between your herb/alcohol mixture and the top of the jar. Place the lid on tightly; affix a label so you know what it is and when it was made. Let the mixture sit for 2 weeks. Shake your tincture every day, while keeping an eye on the alcohol. Make sure there is enough liquid to keep the herbs in solution. If it looks like the herbs have "sucked up" all the alcohol, add enough menstruum to completely cover them again. Make sure this is still the same ratio of 50 percent alcohol and 50 percent water. Fresh herbs that are not completely covered with alcohol can mold. Another tip: I sometimes put a piece of waxed paper between the lid and the jar to make the top easier to remove.

5. After 2 to 4 weeks, line your strainer with muslin, or cheesecloth. Place the lined strainer over a bowl and pour the liquid into the cloth.

6. Squeeze and wring the cloth really hard to get as much of the liquid out as possible. This may be the time to get the strongest person in the house to help out! If you're really serious about making tinctures, there are herbal presses available for purchase. These will generally pull an additional 20 percent of the liquid out of the herbs. I've included suppliers in the resource section.

7. Pour the strained liquid into a dark bottle, label, and store it in a dark cabinet.

8. Compost the leftover herb material in your garden or compost pile to nourish your soil.

Directions for Basic Dried Herb Tincture

Unlike fresh plant, dried herb has no water. Generally, you need 40 to 70 percent alcohol to extract most constituents out of your herb. If you need 50 percent alcohol, the other 50 percent is water. An exception is gums and resins (such as myrrh) that require a solvency of 90 to 95 percent alcohol, and pure grain alcohol is the best option.

1. Take your dried herb, weigh it, and then grind it in your coffee grinder to a fairly consistent coarse powder. "Coarse" is the operative word here. You don't want a fine powder; it's messy to work with.

2. Most tinctures are made in a 1:5 ratio. This means that you'll cover your weighed herb with five times the volume of menstruum. For example, if your herb weighs 50 grams, you will need 250 milliliters (50 x 5 = 250) of solvent.

3. If the solvent required for your herb is 60 percent, this means that roughly 60 percent of the 250 milliliters must be alcohol and 40 percent water (250 x .60 = 150 milliliters). So you would pour 150 milliliters of grain alcohol and 100 milliliters of water over the herb and stir well.

4. Place the lid on tightly; affix a label on the jar so you know what it is and when it was made. Let it sit for 2 to 4 weeks. Shake your tincture every day. Make sure that the liquid completely covers the herbs. If it appears that you need more, then add another 50 milliliters of menstruum to make a 1:6 ratio. Remember, 60 percent of that 50 milliliters needs to be alcohol, the balance water (50 x .60 = 30 milliliters grain alcohol and 20 milliliters water). Stir well. If you still need more alcohol, then add another 50 milliliters of menstruum.

5. After 2 to 4 weeks, line your strainer with muslin, or cheesecloth. Place it over a bowl and pour the liquid into the cloth.
6. Squeeze and wring the cloth really hard to get as much of the liquid out as possible. Once again, get the strongest person in the house to help out. You should be able to get about 150 milliliters of tincture by hand and up to 200 milliliters with a press.
7. Pour strained liquid into a dark bottle, label, and store in a dark cabinet.
8. Compost herbs in your garden or compost pile.

Making tinctures is easy and downright addictive once you get started. Don't be afraid to experiment with different alcohols or alter the taste by adding some dried fruits. Although alcohol is a terrific solvent and preservative, if you are averse to taking it and/or want an alternative for your children, consider using vegetable glycerine to prepare a glycerite.

▶ Herbal Glycerites: Best for Children

Are you falling in love with herbal remedies but cautious about giving them to your children? Don't worry: Glycerin tinctures are a great alternative. They're alcohol-free, because they use vegetable glycerin as a solvent, rather than alcohol. Like alcohol-based tinctures, they are convenient, ready to use whenever or wherever you need them. When my daughter Kiara was colicky as a baby, I would put an eyedropper with chamomile glycerite in the corner of her mouth while I was nursing her. She would just drink it down with my breast milk. It worked like a charm. I also use glycerin tinctures when treating dogs and cats. A favorite is skullcap glycerite, which is very effective for calming highly excitable dogs.

Before we get into the actual instructions for making a glycerite, let's go through some of the basics.

Glycerin is a clear, thick liquid created by hydrolysis of animal or vegetable fats or fixed oils. (I recommend using vegetable glycerin derived from vegetable oil—usually palm—that is readily available at most natural food stores.) Glycerin is sweet and sticky, like a clear sugar, its consistency somewhere between honey and molasses. Glycerin chemically belongs to the "alcohol" group, hence its other name: glycerol. However, it is not an alcohol in the same sense as vodka or brandy. Those who are alcohol-sensitive, are recovering alcoholics, or have liver disease or stomach ulcers may all safely consume vegetable glycerin. Because it is sweet, it makes a good base for kids' medicines and is also safe for use in animals. On the other hand, glycerin does not have the preservative strength of alcohol. If stored well, in dark glass and out of direct sunlight, a glycerite will preserve for two years, maybe a little longer. Although it is a stronger solvent than water, it will not dissolve resins, like those contained in myrrh.

Glycerites are made using the maceration process, described above in the section on making tinctures, pages 38–45. The only difference is that the menstruum is a glycerin/water mixture rather than an alcohol/water mixture.

Glycerites must be made with a minimum of 70 percent glycerin to prevent microbial overgrowth. If you are making a glycerite out of fresh herb, you have to account for the water in the plant, meaning that you have to use almost pure vegetable glycerin.

Glycerin is much more viscous and has a much higher density than alcohol. So, whereas many roots and barks will sink in alcohol, they will tend to float on glycerin; it is often necessary to use a weight (I use pie weights) to make sure that the herb remains covered by the glycerin. For this reason, it is recommended that glycerites be made to a 1:8 ratio specification.

That means if you have 100 grams of herb, you will use 800 milliliters of menstruum, and at least 70 percent of that must be vegetable glycerin.

Directions for Basic Fresh-Herb Glycerite

1. Rinse off any dirt from your herbs, and finely chop them with a knife. Fill a glass jar ¾ full with herbs.
2. Pour enough pure vegetable glycerin to completely cover the herbs and leave an additional 1-inch layer on top. This is important to ensure that uncovered herbs do not get moldy.
3. Take a wooden spoon or chopstick and stir well. Again, make sure that the glycerin completely covers the herb. If desired, you can take a small cloth bag and fill it with ceramic pie weights and drop it down on top of the herbs to weigh them down and keep them from floating to the top.
4. Place the lid on tightly; affix a label on the jar so you know what it is and when it was made. Let it sit for 2 to 4 weeks. Shake your tincture every day or two, keeping an eye on the glycerin. If it looks like the herbs have "sucked up" all the glycerin, add enough to completely cover them again.
5. After 2 to 4 weeks, take your jar of glycerite and put in a pan of water and gently heat, stirring occasionally until the glycerin is thin in consistency. Warming the glycerin makes it easier to strain.
6. Line a strainer with muslin, or cheesecloth. Place the lined strainer over a bowl and carefully pour the warmed liquid into the cloth. (Don't burn yourself!)
7. Squeeze and wring the cloth really hard to get as much of the liquid out as possible.
8. Pour the strained liquid into a dark bottle, label, and store it in a dark cabinet. Your glycerin tincture will remain potent for roughly 2 years.
9. Compost the leftover herb material in your garden or compost pile to nourish your soil.

Basic Directions for Dried-Herb Glycerite

When making a glycerite out of dried herbs, you don't need to account for any water in the plant. The primary calculation here is to make sure you use a menstruum ratio of 1:8, and that at least 70 percent of the menstruum is vegetable glycerin.

1. Weigh your dried herb, and then grind it in your coffee grinder so that you have a fairly consistent coarse powder. "Coarse" is the operative word here. You don't want a fine powder; it's messy to work with.

2. You want to use a 1:8 ratio. This means that you'll cover your weighed herb with eight times the volume of solvent. For example, if your herb weighs 50 grams, you will need 400 milliliters (50 x 8 = 400) of solvent.

3. For glycerites made from dried herb, you need at least 70 percent vegetable glycerin and 30 percent water. So you would multiply 400 x .70 to get 280 milliliters of glycerin and 120 milliliters of water. If you are making a number of glycerites, I recommend mixing up a batch of 70 percent glycerin and 30 percent water and storing in a container. This way, it is already premade in the correct percentage and you just have to pour it over the herb.

4. Cover herbs with the glycerin and water. Place the lid on tightly; affix a label on the jar so you know what it is and when it was made. Let it sit for 2 to 6 weeks. Shake your tincture every day. Make sure that the liquid completely covers the herbs. If it appears that you need more, add another 50 milliliters of solvent to make a 1:9 ratio. Remember, 70 percent of that 50 milliliters needs to be glycerin, the balance water (50 x .70 = 35 milliliters glycerin and 15 milliliters water). Stir well. If you still need more glycerin, then repeat. (This is why I like to premake my glycerin/water blend; I can skip all the calculations and just add another 50 milliliters at a time.)

5. After 2 to 4 weeks, take your jar of glycerite and put it in a pan of water and gently heat, stirring occasionally until the glycerin is thin in consistency.

6. Line a strainer with muslin, or cheesecloth. Place it over a bowl and pour the warmed liquid into the cloth. Squeeze and wring the cloth really hard to get as much of the liquid out as possible.

7. Pour the strained liquid into a dark bottle, label, and store in a dark cabinet. Your glycerite has a shelf life of roughly 2 years.

8. Compost herbs in your garden or compost pile.

Some of my favorite herbs for making glycerites, especially for children and animals, are:

- *Skullcap*. Skullcap is a very safe and gentle herb that I have used in clinical practice and at home for many years. In the early 1980s, skullcap got a bad and undeserved reputation, with claims that it caused liver damage. Not true. Studies found that the problem was due to adulteration with germander (*Teucrium* spp.), a totally unrelated plant. The *Botanical Safety Handbook*, 2nd edition, gives skullcap a safety rating of 1A, meaning there are no known safety issues or precautions with use.

- *Chamomile*. If you have children, chamomile glycerite is one remedy you should definitely make and keep on hand. This remedy is widely known for its ability to relieve indigestion, colic, intestinal cramping, and nausea, while calming the most unhappy toddler. But chamomile isn't only for children; it's also amazing for adults.

- *Barberry*. Like goldenseal and Oregon grape root, barberry *(Berberis vulgaris)* is high in berberine, a yellow-colored alkaloid that has a wide range of activity against numerous bacteria, fungi, and parasites.

▶ Oils and Salves: Herbal Must-Haves

As a massage therapist, I made countless gallons of herbal massage oils to ease sore muscles and promote relaxation. As an herbalist and physician, I've made gallons of salves to alleviate eczema, soothe psoriasis, treat athlete's foot and skin irritations, and heal minor cuts and scrapes. As a mother, I've relied on herbal oils and salves to soothe all kinds of boo-boos and, of course, as a chef, I delight in gathering fresh herbs from my garden and making infused oils for cooking. And for me personally, I find few things more delightful than infusing lavender in grape seed or almond oil and adding it to my bath at the end of a long day. Infused oils are wonderful additions to both the kitchen cupboard and the medicine pantry.

Learning to make an infused oil or herbal salve is relatively easy. Let's go over a few of the basics to get your started.

Fixed, or fatty, oils are so called because they are not volatile, meaning they are not highly combustible nor do they evaporate. They are liquid at room temperature and are insoluble in water. You've probably used numerous fixed oils in your kitchen: olive, safflower, sunflower, almond, apricot kernel, walnut, grape seed, and more. They are the solvent of choice for massage oils, and make an excellent base for salves. Herbalists and massage practitioners often have very pronounced preferences as to which oils are "best"; however, the oils may be pretty much used interchangeably. Just make sure you store your oil in a dark cool place, as prolonged exposure to high heat or light will turn them rancid.

Essential oils are volatile aromatic compounds derived from plants, typically through steam distillation. These highly concentrated oils are used in perfumery, soaps, flavorings, aromatherapy, and of course, in herbal medicine. Many have powerful antiseptic and anti-inflammatory activity, making them highly useful in medicinal salves. High-quality essential oils can be costly but you only need to use a very small amount in your preparations. Examples of commonly used essential oils include tea tree oil for acne, and fungal, yeast, and bacterial infections; eucalyptus oil for sinus congestion, insect stings, and muscle pain; lavender oil for skin inflammation, sore muscles, and anxiety; and peppermint essential oil for congestion, headache, muscle tension, aches, and pains.

You will also find me and others using the terms "carrier oil" and "infused oil." Carrier oil is essentially another name for a fixed oil that has been used to dilute or "carry" essential oils before applying to the skin. An infused oil is simply a fixed oil that has been infused with one or more herbs.

A salve, also called an ointment or unguent, is a semisolid fatty preparation that is used externally on the skin. In herbal medicine, salves are primarily made using infused oils for the base with beeswax to thicken and harden the salve. Salves can also be made from animal fat (for example, lard), but this practice is much less common today.

Sometimes tincture of benzoin, vitamin E, or an essential oil is added to a salve to enhance its preservation. Most salves do fine without these if they are kept at a stable temperature in a tightly lidded container.

Directions for Basic Herb-Infused Oil

1. Fill a quart glass jar ¾ full with dried herb, preferably freshly dried.
2. Cover herbs with a fixed oil, filling the jar to within an inch of the top. You can choose whatever oil you'd like. Many people use olive, grape seed, or almond oil.
3. Cover with a tight-fitting lid and label the lid or jar with the name of the herb and the date it was prepared.
4. Place the jar in a paper bag and set out in the sun or in a sunny place. You want the heat, not the light.
5. Shake your oil every day for 2 to 4 weeks. Top off with more oil if needed. You want the herb to be completely covered by the oil.

6. Layer a strainer with cheesecloth or muslin and place the cloth over a large bowl.
7. Pour the contents of the jar into a strainer and squeeze to get as much oil out as possible. Set the remaining herbs aside for composting in your garden.
8. Pour the infused oil into a bottle, cap or cork tightly, and label it. If stored in a cool, dark place, the oil will stay good for at least a year. If possible, store in your refrigerator or root cellar.

Some of my favorite herbs for making infused oils:

- *Arnica.* This herb is an absolute essential for any busy family. I use both arnica tincture and arnica oil on a regular basis. It is a powerhouse anti-inflammatory and analgesic, easing the pain of bruises, strains, sprains, and arthritic joints. Arnica should not be used on broken skin; it's for topical use only. I usually combine equal parts of arnica oil with St. John's wort oil.
- *German chamomile flowers.* These make a wonderful salve. A number of scientific studies have shown that chamomile creams and ointments relieve eczema as effectively as low-potency hydrocortisone without any of the side effects that can come with using topical steroids.
- *Chaparral leaf.* This herb is a traditional wound healer down in the southwestern part of the United States. A slow-growing desert dweller, chaparral possesses powerful antifungal, antibacterial, and anti-inflammatory activity. I often include it in my all-purpose wound salves.
- *Comfrey root.* Here you have one of the most revered herbal wound medicines. It relieves pain and inflammation and can be used for burns, insect bites, and skin irritation. Scientific studies have shown that comfrey ointment can alleviate back pain when applied topically. Comfrey

contains allantoin, a compound shown to increase cell proliferation, hence its name *Symphytum,* from the Greek *symphyo,* meaning to "make grow together," for its renown as a wound healer. Comfrey contains trace amounts of pyrrolizidine alkaloids, compounds that can damage the liver if taken in sufficient quantities. To be on the safe side, only use comfrey topically.

- *Goldenseal root.* This herb is an indigenous North American plant that has been used for centuries for treating wounds. One of its chief constituents is berberine, an alkaloid that possesses significant antimicrobial activity against a wide range of harmful bacteria. I don't generally use goldenseal because it has been so overharvested. Make sure to buy it organically grown, but it's expensive. I use barberry root bark and Oregon grape root with excellent results. I couldn't imagine taking care of all the cuts and scrapes over the years without them.

- *Mullein flowers.* Steeped in olive oil, mullein flowers are a luscious and soothing remedy for ear infections. This oil can be used by itself or blended with garlic oil for ear infections, as well as to treat mite infections in dogs. Toward the end of every summer, I make a fresh small batch. If I'm not busy, I'll make the mullein oil in olive oil, let it set for 2 weeks, and then strain the oil and pour it over a whole new jar of mullein flowers. I'll repeat that 2 to 3 times to make it stronger. Mullein magic.

- *St. John's wort.* Here is one of the most beautiful oils you'll ever make. A deep, ruby-colored oil that is marvelous for easing the pain of sciatica, shingles, or other types of nerve pain. When the beautiful yellow St. John's wort flowers are blooming, cut the flowering tops, the upper 3 to 4 inches of the plant, in late morning, and let them wilt overnight to remove some of the moisture. Then make your infused oil.

Healing Herbal Salves

A salve is simple to make, especially if you have an array of infused oils on hand. Elsewhere in this book I've given recipes for making some blended salves—BUT I strongly encourage you to make your infused oils individually. Then you can blend them together in whatever ways you wish for salve or to use as massage or body oil. Just blend together in the amounts you want and use roughly 2 ounces grated beeswax for every 8 ounces of infused oil.

Herbal salves can be used as a first aid remedy or carried in your purse for chapped lips. Of course, I've been known to use lard, lanolin, cocoa butter, and other bases—but follow this basic recipe using a beeswax base for a straightforward and easy way to make salves.

Basic Directions for Herbal Salve

1. Pour 8 ounces of infused herbal oil into the top of a double boiler. If you don't have a double boiler, you can use a saucepan, but just make sure to keep it on very low heat to avoid burning the oil.

2. Grate your beeswax using an inexpensive cheese grater. It's easier to use when grated and melts more quickly. Just be prepared to essentially donate the cheese grater to your salve-making equipment, as the beeswax is a pain to clean off! For that matter, your spatula or wooden spoon should probably be relegated to the same collection.

3. Add 2 ounces of beeswax to the oil and gently melt, stirring frequently. The tricky part is getting the salve to the right consistency. Dip a spoon into the mixture and put it on a paper towel and stick it in your refrigerator for 5 minutes. Take it out. If it's mushy, add 1 to 2 tablespoons more grated beeswax. If it's too hard (not likely, but possible) add 2 to 3 tablespoons of extra infused oil. Repeat this process until you get it to the right consistency. Bottom line: too mushy—needs more beeswax; too hard—needs more infused oil.

R℞ PRESCRIPTION FROM DR. LOW DOG
Infused Oils in a Hurry

If you need an herbal oil or salve and don't have 2 to 4 weeks to wait, take the following shortcut and make what you need in an afternoon. Granted, these remedies aren't quite as strong, but they certainly will work if you're pinched for time.

Fill your jar with the herb and cover with oil, just as we did previously. This time, though, dump the entire jar into the top of your double boiler, and turn the heat on the lowest setting. Cover the pan, and cook on very low temperature for 1 to 2 hours. Stir frequently to prevent scorching the oil. Strain out the herb and, voilà—you now have an infused oil that you can use as is, or as a base for salve.

If using fresh herbs, it's best to cook the herbs in a Crock-Pot on the lowest setting, with the lid off, for 8 to 10 hours. Start it in the morning and let it go all day. Stir frequently, and don't scorch the oil or stop too soon, or you'll have water in the oil. Strain out the herbs and use as is or as a base for salve.

---

4. Remove the pan from the heat. If desired, add some vitamin E and/or essential oils. I like to add natural vitamin E (d-alpha tocopherol), because it's so nice on the skin and it helps stabilize the oil. You can purchase this online or in most health food stores. You can use an essential oil as an addition, or instead of vitamin E. To prevent sensitivity to the essential oil, stick with 1 to 2 percent essential oil dilution. For a 1 percent dilution, add 6 drops per fluid ounce of infused oil. For a 2 percent dilution, add 12 drops per fluid ounce of infused oil. Just remember, vitamin E and/or essential oils need to be added at the very end to avoid prolonged exposure to heat.

5. Stir well and pour into salve containers or tins. Let them sit for 1 to 2 hours, until the salve is completely hardened. Place lids on the tins or glass jars and label.

Chapter 2

Understanding and Managing Infections

Infection is one of the most common problems encountered by all members of the household. Ranging from the mild but annoying cold and upper respiratory infection, to the potentially dangerous pneumonia or nephritis (kidney infection)—it is important to be able to distinguish between the minor and self-limited infections and those that can be deadly if not properly treated. Even minor infections can turn dangerous in young infants and elders if you aren't paying attention. I will be discussing infections in other chapters of this book as they relate to the skin, gastrointestinal and respiratory systems, and bladder—still, I feel like it's important to start with some background and guidelines for treating these problems at home. This is especially true when it comes to treating children, elders, and those whose immune systems may be weakened due to illness or medication.

What Causes Infections

Infections are caused by microbes—organisms too small to see with the naked eye. Microbes can be divided into basically four groups: bacteria, viruses, fungi, or protozoa. Bacteria are single-celled microorganisms that exist almost everywhere in the environment, from the extreme cold in Antarctica to places with very high temperatures like hot springs and volcanoes. Bacteria also inhabit the human body. The *Lactobacilli* that live in our gastrointestinal tract help aid in the digestion of food and the production of vitamins, and help fend off dangerous bacteria and even help fight cancer. The vast majority of bacteria are not harmful. In fact, less than one percent of bacteria cause disease in human beings. However, some can be very dangerous. The bubonic plague that killed roughly one-third of the people living in Europe during the 14th century was caused by *Yersinia pestis,* a bacterium that spreads through fleas. We still see cases of bubonic plague occasionally in New Mexico. More common bacterial infections include urinary tract infections, strep throat, and certain skin infections.

Viruses are smaller than bacteria and consist only of molecules of RNA or DNA surrounded by a protein coat. Unlike bacteria, most viruses cause disease. Between 1918 and 1919, the influenza virus killed roughly 20 million people around the world, while the human immunodeficiency virus, which causes AIDS, has taken the lives of more than 2 million. Viruses differ from other microbes in that they cannot survive without a host. The virus invades a healthy cell and, once inside, reprograms the host cell to reproduce more viral particles, until the cell eventually dies. Viruses cause many common infections such as colds, flu, most coughs and bronchitis, and roughly 80 to 90 percent of sore throats.

A fungus is basically a primitive plant. Hundreds of thousands of different fungi share our world and most are not harmful to us. Certain mushrooms have long been enjoyed as a food, yeasts are used to ferment foods and make bread, and molds have been transformed into antibiotics like penicillin. When a fungus causes disease, it is called mycoses. Common mycoses infections

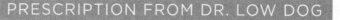

R̲x̲ PRESCRIPTION FROM DR. LOW DOG

Microbes Associated With Common Infections

Condition	Bacteria	Virus	Fungus	Protozoa
Athlete's foot			X	
Bladder infection	X			
Colds		X		
Diarrhea	X	X		X
Ear infection	X	X	X	
Flu		X		
Herpes		X		
Lyme disease	X			
Pneumonia	X	X	X	
Sinusitis	X		X	
Skin disease	X	X	X	X
Strep throat	X			
Vaginal infection	X		X	X
Whooping cough	X			

include athlete's foot and ringworm, which I will discuss in the chapter on skin.

Protozoa are microscopic one-celled animals. Plankton is a type of protozoa that serves as food for whales and other marine life. However, when protozoa invade the human body, they generally cause disease. They are generally transmitted either by ingesting contaminated food or water, or by being bitten by mosquitoes or sand flies. *Plasmodium falciparum* is one of the most virulent species of protozoa that causes malaria and is transmitted by mosquitoes. Roughly 250 million people around the world are infected. *Giardia* is a major cause of diarrheal disease around the world, infecting up to one-third of people living in developing countries. It is the most common intestinal parasitic disease in the United States. *Giardia* is found in soil, food, or water that has been contaminated with the feces of infected humans or animals.

The Body's Defenses

Because human beings have evolved with the trillions of microbes that also share our world, our bodies are extremely well designed to keep us from getting sick. Your skin provides a strong physical barrier. The mucus in your nose and lungs, and small hairlike structures called cilia, trap microbes. Coughing and sneezing then help the mucus move those germs out of your body more efficiently. Your stomach's powerful stomach acid can destroy most disease-causing microorganisms. Healthy bacteria live on our skin and within our digestive tract, competing with harmful bacteria for nutrients. Even your sweat and tears contain lysozymes, or enzymes that inhibit bacterial growth! Of course, this is why you don't want to interfere too much with nature's design. Taking medications that shut down stomach acid long-term is not a good idea because it increases your risk for infection, as well as making it difficult for you to absorb critical immune-enhancing nutrients. Broad-spectrum antibiotics destroy both good and bad bacteria, leaving the body with fewer natural defenses.

But if some sneaky bacteria or parasite manages to get past all of these initial defenses, you have an exquisite immune system designed to keep you healthy. You have a fast-acting rapid-response team (cell-mediated immunity), and a long-term strategic defense group (antibody-mediated immunity). As a matter of fact, the body is so well designed for staving off infections that a growing body of research shows that if the immune system isn't challenged during early childhood, it can actually begin to work against us, seeing harmless things, like pollen, cat hair, or gluten, as foreign invaders. It may even view cells within our own body as dangerous, leading to autoimmune diseases.

There's no question we're seeing increasing rates of allergies and autoimmune diseases in developed nations, and medical scientists are linking this to the excessive use of antibiotics in children, fewer people living on farms and lack of early exposure to animals, and a growing number of babies being born by Cesarean section, which alters and delays the development of healthy gut microflora. What I'm trying to say is that getting dirty, catching colds, and playing with puppies are all good for training the immune system to understand what is harmful and what is safe. I have long considered it a good day when the children came home with grass in their hair and mud on their pants.

Antibiotics and Resistance

Although our bodies are well suited for preventing and dealing with infections, some pathogens can be very dangerous, and some members of our population may be particularly vulnerable. There can be little debate that one gift of modern medicine has been the development of antibiotics that can treat serious infection. As a physician, I've seen many patients admitted to the hospital with a severe infection in their lungs, blood, or kidneys who, after just a few days of receiving the proper antibiotic treatment, walked out of the hospital well on their way to health. Because I have such deep respect for the power of antibiotics, I am concerned about the growing number of antibiotic-resistant microorganisms that have become part of our modern landscape. A study published in 2012 in the Centers for Disease Control journal found that the proportion of *Escherichia coli* bacteria that have developed multidrug resistance had increased from 7.2 percent during the 1950s to 63.6 percent during the

2000s. This means that at least three major classes of antibiotics were ineffective for treating *E. coli,* a bacterium associated with GI infections, urinary tract infections, and meningitis.

When people are infected with a drug-resistant organism, they often require treatment with second- or third-choice antibiotics that may be less effective and more toxic. With the world becoming increasingly interconnected through trade and travel, the ability for resistant microorganisms to spread rapidly to distant countries and continents is now a sobering reality. Antibiotic resistance is due, in part, to the overprescribing of antibiotics for minor infections that would be much better suited to home treatment and natural medicines. Antibiotics are routinely given to those with colds, ear infections, and other viral infections that are not responsive to these drugs.

This rests both on the clinicians' and patients' shoulders, as I experienced nights at the emergency room when it was hard not to pull out the prescription pad when a parent was pleading with me to give her child an antibiotic. Single-parent families are the norm in the United States, and the sad reality is that many cannot afford to stay home nursing a sick child, or worse, are required by their employer and/or child's school to show a doctor's note attesting to an illness. This drives up doctor visits and invariably increases the likelihood of inappropriate prescribing.

If your clinician does recommend an antibiotic, ask if it is necessary. Are there other things you can try for 24 to 48 hours before filling the prescription? And if you decide that taking the antibiotic makes sense, it's vitally important that you take it exactly as directed. People will often stop taking their medication early because they feel better, but the problem is this: The bacteria that survive can become drug-resistant, making the medication ineffective the next time it is prescribed. This increases the likelihood that the infection will continue to smolder inside, and that the most effective drug will be less likely to work. Take-home message: Take your antibiotics for the duration they are prescribed.

Another reason for this growing antibiotic resistance that few people seem to be talking about is the indiscriminate use of antibiotics in livestock and poultry. Inhumane, industrialized animal practices require antibiotics to be given early and often to prevent epidemic infections and promote growth in overcrowded environments. Researchers in the United States and Europe have now found close genetic matches between resistant *E. coli* found in human urine and resistant strains found on chicken and turkey sold in supermarkets. Foodborne urinary tract infections, as they are now known, are a growing problem. When raw poultry meat is improperly handled, bacteria take up residence in the gastrointestinal tract until the time is ripe for infection. Both organic and conventionally grown chickens are commonly contaminated with *E. coli.*

In fact, in 2010, the National Antimicrobial Resistance Monitoring System (NARMS) reported that more than 75 percent of chicken and turkey, 59 percent of ground beef, and 40 percent of pork products tested in the United States were contaminated with *E. coli,* and that a large portion of this foodborne *E. coli* was multidrug-resistant (to three or more classes of antibiotics). It is SO important to wash utensils, as well as your hands, that have come into contact with raw meats. Vegetables and fruits can also harbor harmful bacteria, so always wash your produce, even when it says "prewashed." Safe food practices are one important step you can take to protect the health of you and your family.

Antibiotic resistance is a serious problem for everyone. With every introduction of a new antibiotic into the marketplace, resistant strains of bacteria are detected within just a few years, and at this time, there are virtually no new antibiotics in the drug pipeline. We must all be better educated about preventing infection, as well as learning to distinguish when antibiotics are needed and when we can make do without them. In each section of this chapter, I will provide you with the information you need to discern the difference.

Prevention Is in Your Hands

We all know that one of the most effective ways to prevent infectious illness is to wash our hands. That's because the vast majority of microbes are transmitted from your hands to your nose and mouth. You should always wash your hands after using the bathroom, changing a diaper, before preparing or eating food, and whenever you are caring for someone who is sick. You do not need to use antibacterial soap. I'm not a fan of most of these products, as many contain triclosan, a chemical linked to liver damage, decreased thyroid function, and muscle weakness. Plus, I'm concerned that overuse of antibacterial soaps is contributing to the growing problem with bacterial resistance.

According to the Centers for Disease Control (CDC), antibacterial-containing products have not been proven to prevent the spread of infection better than products that do not contain antibacterial chemicals. In other words, plain soap and water work just fine! So just soap up and wash your hands for

Homemade Foaming Soap

1 cup water
1/3 cup liquid castile soap
5 drops essential oil (optional)
Soap bottle with foaming pump

Put the water and liquid castile soap into a soap bottle with a foaming pump, and you are good to go. It's that simple. If you don't want it to foam, just use a soap bottle with a regular pump. You can give yourself a little extra protection naturally by adding 5 drops of your favorite essential oil. Citrus is really nice for the kitchen, while lavender or peppermint are great for the bathroom. Liquid castile soap can be purchased online and in many health food stores. I love the old classic Dr. Bronner's organic castile soap.

15 seconds. I taught my kids to sing the happy birthday song, which is about—you guessed it—15 seconds long.

Immune Boosters

A healthy body is well positioned to fend off harmful microbes. But are there things you can do to actually "boost" your immune response or help stave off harmful microbes? Many traditional systems of medicine had special herbs and/or foods that were recommended to help keep the body strong and reduce the risk of infection. Garlic, onions, and leeks have long been recommended, and modern science shows that they may indeed help keep you from catching a cold or getting diarrhea.

If you seem to catch everything that goes around your school or office, I would suggest you consider taking a basic multivitamin that provides 15 to 20 milligrams of zinc and 200 to 400 milligrams of vitamin C for extra infection-fighting nutrients. Both of these nutrients are critically important for optimal functioning of the immune system. Studies have shown that healthy children who take zinc regularly have fewer colds, fewer school absences, and less antibiotic use. Taking vitamin C regularly can shorten the duration of colds by about 8 percent in adults and 14 percent in children.

Astragalus membranaceus, also known as *huang qi,* is native to northern China and is considered one of the most important herbs in traditional Chinese medicine. It is taken to strengthen the immune system and prevent upper respiratory infections. Scientific studies support this. Astragalus increases immune cells in nasal secretions, one of your first lines of defense against respiratory infections. It also can rev up your "rapid-response" team of T cells, making your body better able to fight off an infection if it gains a foothold. Astragalus is quite safe. In China, a few pieces of the dried root are cooked in soups, especially during the wet and/or cold times of the year.

For a real immune boost, you could include some medicinal mushrooms in your meals a couple times a week or take a supplement. Although mushrooms have many compounds that contribute to their beneficial effects on human health, it is the polysaccharides, large complex carbohydrates that account for their potent antiviral and immune-enhancing properties. Mushroom polysaccharides have been scientifically shown to help the body resist infection and fight off tumor cells, making them an excellent addition to the diet any time of year, but especially during the long cold winter months. Here are three of my favorites.

Shiitake *(Lentinus edodes)* is a culinary mushroom enjoyed around the world for its delicious meaty taste. Shiitake are highly nutritious, being a good source of vitamins B_2, B_5, B_6; iron, magnesium, vitamin D_2, and protein. It contains lentinan, a polysaccharide with potent immune-boosting and antiviral activity.

Maitake *(Grifola frondosa)*, or "dancing mushroom" in Japanese, is another culinary mushroom that can be enjoyed raw,

Simply Shiitake

2 cups fresh shiitake mushrooms, stemmed and sliced
2 cloves garlic
2 green onions, chopped
2 tablespoons olive oil
1 tablespoon light brown sugar
1 tablespoon lemon juice
1 tablespoon tamari or low-sodium soy sauce

Remove stems and slice shiitake into $1/2$-inch pieces. Crush garlic and let sit for 10 minutes; this allows the medicinal benefits to be released so that the garlic can be heated. Mix the lemon juice, tamari, and brown sugar. Heat the oil in a skillet and cook mushrooms for 5 minutes. Add garlic and sauté for 1 to 2 minutes. Add the tamari mixture and cook until absorbed. Remove from heat. Top with chopped green onion and, if desired, a few drops of dark sesame oil. Serve as a side dish or over rice, chicken, or fish.

roasted, grilled, baked, or sautéed. It is a good source of B vitamins, vitamin D, and protein, and a mere 3 ounces provide almost 1,000 IU of vitamin D_2!

You may have also heard of reishi *(Ganoderma lucidum)*. Only the hard core will want to attempt to eat this very tough fibrous mushroom. It's strictly a medicinal mushroom in my book. But with more than 400 bioactive compounds and a large body of evidence confirming its immune-enhancing, anti-inflammatory, anticancer, and cardiovascular benefits, this is one mushroom you might want to take as a supplement.

The Power of Garlic

People have long believed that garlic can help ward off colds, infections, and of course vampires. While I'm not so sure about the vampires, I can say with confidence that adding garlic to your diet can certainly help you maintain a healthy respiratory and digestive tract, two areas that are vulnerable to infection. On the next page you'll find one of my family's favorite ways of taking garlic.

The Power of Probiotics

Probiotics (a term that means "favoring life") are healthy bacteria that normally inhabit the vagina and intestinal tract and are important for keeping harmful bacteria from wreaking havoc. Yogurt and oral probiotic supplements are good sources of these beneficial bacteria. Yogurts that say "live and active cultures" contain beneficial bacteria (probiotics) that help defend against harmful invaders. Fermented foods like sauerkraut, kefir, or miso soup have been part of the cuisine of traditional cultures for millennia. These foods are rich in prebiotics, substances that provide nourishment for the beneficial bacteria in your GI system. Regular intakes of these "live foods" and their associated bacteria definitely have positive effects on our overall health.

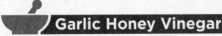
Garlic Honey Vinegar

1 cup (8 ounces) apple cider vinegar, organic and raw preferred
1 tablespoon fennel seed
1 tablespoon fresh ginger, grated
1 small onion, chopped
8 cloves garlic, crushed and let sit for 10 minutes
1 cup (8 ounces) honey, local if possible

Put the apple cider vinegar in a saucepan and add fennel seed and grated ginger. Simmer on very low heat, covered, for 10 minutes. Turn off the heat and let sit for 10 minutes. While this is steeping, crush the garlic and let it sit for 10 minutes, allowing key enzymes to activate the medicinal components in the garlic. If you heat garlic before this enzymatic action takes place, you will lose most of its health benefits. Chop the onion and add it and the garlic to the liquid in the saucepan. Cover and steep for 60 minutes. Strain. Pour the liquid back into a clean saucepan and add the honey. Gently stir on very low heat. Pour into a glass jar and store in the refrigerator; this will keep for months.

How to Use: Use it to dress vegetables, salads, or meat dishes. As medicine, take 1 tablespoon every 3 to 4 hours when you're coming down with the sniffles or dealing with diarrhea.

Garlic, as well as onions, help to protect the gastrointestinal tract from damage when eaten as part of your regular diet. What's more, garlic has been dubbed Russian penicillin because it has been widely used in folk medicine to ward off colds and respiratory and intestinal infections. Raw apple cider vinegar is made from whole apples and is rich in minerals, nutritious, and great for the digestion and intestinal microflora. I absolutely love this garlic honey vinegar as food and medicine.

There is a very large and growing body of evidence that probiotics can be used to prevent and treat gastrointestinal infections and prevent antibiotic-induced diarrhea. Antibiotics are notorious for altering your inner ecology and decimating the vaginal and intestinal tracts of good bacteria. Probiotics restore and maintain the balance between good and bad bacteria in your body. They also give you an edge against bladder infections by preventing the growth of nasty microbes, such as *Escherichia coli,* one of the main bacteria responsible for urinary tract infections.

I always recommend that my patients take a probiotic while taking antibiotics to reduce the risk of antibiotic-associated diarrhea and yeast infection. The following strains of probiotics have been clinically shown to be effective at the doses provided and can be found in many pharmacies and almost all health food stores/natural grocers. Take these at least two hours apart from the antibiotic and continue to take them for seven days after completing your treatment.

For children up to 12 years of age:
- *Saccharomyces boulardii:* 250 milligrams 2 times a day
- *Lactobacillus* GG: 1 billion colony-forming units 1 time a day

For people 12 years and older:
- *Saccharomyces boulardii:* 500 milligrams 2 times a day
- *Lactobacillus* GG: 1 billion colony-forming units 2 times a day

◆ Special Concerns: Children and Infection

Children are going to get sick. There will be numerous colds and upper respiratory infections, bouts of diarrhea and vomiting, and any number of bumps, cuts, and bruises. As I mentioned previously, this is in no small part how their immune system is stretched, worked out, and trained to respond appropriately. As a physician and a mother, I have cared for many sick children over the past three decades. I took hundreds of "mommy" calls in the middle of the night, helping parents decide if they should bring their child into the urgent care or wait until morning. I remember one lovely young mother who was so distraught over her child's fever and cough that I told her to bring her down to the emergency room, as the urgent care had already closed. When I went in to see them, I saw this adorable red-cheeked little 20-month-old girl climbing around on the gurney grabbing at the blood pressure cuff, and then at my stethoscope, fussing to get down and run around. I offered her a graham cracker and a small cup of apple juice, which she got down without difficulty. I examined her, and other than a stuffy nose, mildly red right ear, and fever of 101°F, she was fine. I reassured mom that her child was going to be fine and that her child's body was doing exactly what it was supposed to, and told her what to look for as far as symptoms that would be concerning.

When I asked if she had anyone to help out at home or a relative nearby, she told me it was just her and her little girl after the father left. Her family was more than a thousand miles away. She had no grandparent around to offer advice, no aunt or older sister with children who could help guide her. Trust me, when an elder grandmother told me she was worried about a young child, I almost always said to bring the baby in. As our communities become more dispersed and isolated, it is harder for young parents to find a trusted source for advice, other than what they can Google late at night. Maybe this is why I've always loved teaching early parenting classes. Those who attend are so hungry for information and so appreciative for what they learn. That's another reason I chose to write this book, to help reach those that I cannot personally see.

As you go through the following sections, if your baby is more than two months old, sick, and the following statements are true . . .

- Your child continues to drink fluids
- Your child is eating some food, even if it is less than normal
- Your infant is having six or more wet diapers a day
- Your child is peeing regularly every few hours
- Your child has tears when she cries

- Despite feeling bad, your child is interactive
- You are able to awaken your child when sleeping

. . . then it is highly likely that you can treat your child safely at home. To a physician, these are all highly reassuring signs that your child is doing OK. If your child is doing all of these, then the following do not warrant an immediate trip to the urgent care or emergency room, but you should definitely call your child's health care provider for:

- A fever of 103°F or higher in a child under the age of three, or *any* fever lasting longer than three days in a child of any age
- Lack of improvement if you're treating a minor ailment and nothing seems to make it better within five days, or it worsens
- Thick eye discharge that sticks the eyelid together and doesn't get better during the day
- Exposure to a contagious disease such as mono, whooping cough, measles, or flu, or illness after recently traveling out of the country

It is just as important to know the "danger" signs for a child who has an infection. As a physician, I am highly concerned if your child has any of the symptoms in the following list, and I would strongly recommend that you take your child immediately to the nearest emergency room or urgent care.

➕ **Seek Medical Attention Now for a Child With an Infection**

- When a baby under two months of age (one exception is if your two-month-old just got her vaccinations and runs a low-grade fever within 36 hours) has a rectal temperature of 100.4°F or higher

- When the sudden onset of any fever is accompanied by pain in one leg or joint
- When a high fever with a red rash remains colored after you press down on it (could indicate a serious infection, including meningitis, a dangerous infection in the tissues surrounding the brain)
- When a fever is accompanied by a stiff neck and extreme lack of energy (could be meningitis)
- When any pain is persistent or worsens (such as ear pain, headache, or sore throat), despite the use of over-the-counter pain relievers and/or natural medicines
- When a child of any age has severe abdominal pain, or pain in the belly that is worsened when the child jumps up and down (could indicate appendicitis or intestinal obstruction)
- When diarrhea is bloody or there is blood in the vomit, which can indicate a severe infection. (Children may have a little bright blood in their stool from tiny anal tears that come from straining a firm/hard stool—this is not an emergency.)
- When an infant has a stool that looks like grape or currant jelly (this could indicate an intestinal obstruction)
- When there is difficulty breathing, wheezing, or labored or noisy breathing
- When there is an inability to keep down enough fluids to pee at least once every six hours while awake, or if an infant doesn't have a wet diaper in eight hours. (Dehydration is dangerous for young children—see the section in Chapter 5 on Diarrhea, pages 185–193, for strategies for preventing it.)

◗ Special Concerns: Elders and Infection

One evening, I took care of an 82-year-old woman who was brought to the emergency room at the University of New Mexico hospital. Her daughter told me that her mom had stopped eating, was sleeping more, and she'd become very confused that evening. The daughter wasn't sure what was wrong with her because she didn't seem to have a fever or seem sick.

It turned out that this elder woman had a severe bladder infection that had made its way into her kidneys and then her bloodstream. She had no temperature and hadn't noticed any signs of a urinary tract infection. What's more, the laboratory tests that check for white blood cells (immune cells) had come back normal. We admitted her to the hospital, and I'm happy to report that she recovered and was discharged within a few days because she received the appropriate intravenous antibiotics and fluids.

This collection of "nonsymptoms" may seem odd, but truth be told, I've cared for many elders who were very sick but lacked most or all of the signs that we'd normally see in someone younger. Elders often fail to exhibit typical symptoms of illness or infection, so it's very important to err on the side of caution when it comes to those who are 75 years of age and older. When something doesn't "feel right," trust your intuition and make sure you seek proper medical care. It's normal for our immune system to weaken with advancing age. That's why one of the cardinal signs that normally alert us to the presence of an infection—fever—is highly unreliable in elders.

Pay particular attention to prevention with elders. The most common sites for infection are their urinary and respiratory tracts, and the skin. Staying well hydrated, taking cranberry tablets, and maintaining good hygiene can help reduce the risk of bladder infections. Consider pneumonia and/or flu vaccinations, particularly if there is any underlying heart or respiratory disease that could make getting these illnesses dangerous. Keep the skin moisturized. Dry skin is more likely to crack or tear, providing an opening for bacteria to enter. Virgin coconut oil is a great moisturizer and also has natural antibacterial properties.

Seek Medical Attention Now for an Elder With an Infection

I cannot say this too often, or in too many ways: *Always err on the side of caution.* It is NEVER wrong to call your health care provider or go to the urgent care/emergency room for help. Early assessment by a trained health care professional and appropriate treatment is crucial for addressing infections in our elders. You should seek medical attention when there is:

- Fever of 101.5°F or higher in someone over the age of 65
- An acute change in behavior or daily activities
- Increased confusion
- New onset or worsening dizziness
- Fatigue or lethargy
- Loss of appetite
- Red or inflamed area of the skin
- New onset of incontinence or increased urination
- Blood in the urine
- Shortness of breath
- New onset or increased pain
- New or change in cough

◗ Other Special Groups: Take Note

Natural medicines are designed to help support your body's own healing process, and that presumes that there is not a genetic or medical condition that suppresses your immune system. Anyone who has been told that they are immune-compromised because of disease or due to medications should not treat any type of infection at home. It is important that you talk to your health care provider to see if you need antibiotics or other supportive therapy if you fall into any of the following categories:

- Are undergoing cancer treatment
- Are taking medications that suppress your immune system, such as medications for autoimmune disease or prednisone

- Have a serious underlying chronic illness, such as heart failure, or kidney or liver disease
- Are pregnant with a fever of 101°F or higher

► Running Hot and Cold: Managing Fever

My daughter was nine months old when she spiked her first 105°F temperature. It was scary. Her entire body felt like it was on fire. I dressed her lightly and gave her some children's Tylenol. Four hours later, the temperature hadn't budged. She wasn't eating or drinking, just sleeping.

After about eight hours of this, I took her over to the University of New Mexico hospital where I was doing my medical training and asked that the pediatric team examine her. Although they gave her ibuprofen and Tylenol, her temperature still hovered right around 105°F. The nurses drew vials of blood. She had a catheter inserted into her bladder to make sure her urine wasn't infected. Swabs were inserted into the back of her nose to check for viral infections.

Poked and prodded for about two hours, my baby girl was hysterical. The team wanted to admit her to the hospital, but because we lived only a few blocks away, I insisted on taking her home to reduce her exposure to other sick children. I remember thinking "she looks so small." The next day, her temperature was hanging out between 103° and 104°F. Her laboratory reports suggested a viral infection. About 48 hours after it all started, her fever broke, her appetite returned, and she was soon back to normal.

About six months later, we went through the same thing all over again but this time I didn't take her to the hospital. I had this sense that Kiara was one of those children who burn hot when they get sick because of a very rigorous immune response. I called the hospital and told them I wouldn't be coming in and settled in for what I knew would be a long day and night. Her temp was close to 105°F. I took off everything but her T-shirt and diaper. I alternated giving her little drinks of chamomile tea sweetened with honey and homemade chicken broth every hour or two. She'd fall sleep, and I'd wake her up to give her the liquids. I didn't give her the immune herb echinacea because I figured her immune system knew what it was doing and didn't need any help. I was calmer this time; we'd done this dance before.

The next day, her temp was staying close to 102°F, and within 72 hours, her temperature was normal.

I tell this story because I know how scary high fevers can be. In my practice, I cannot count the number of parents who've brought their children in, or called me in the middle of the night, because they watched that fever climb and didn't know what to do. A high fever almost always means infection, and that can be worrisome. But it's important to remember that fever is the body's way of defending itself.

When our immune cells encounter a harmful bacteria or virus (pathogens), chemicals called pyrogens are released. Pyrogens, literally meaning "fire producing," travel to the temperature-regulating center in the brain, telling it to raise the body's thermostat. To generate heat, your muscles shiver and you start reaching for the blankets because you feel cold. Sometimes the body "overshoots" the mark, and you feel hot and sweaty, which acts to cool the body to reach the temperature set by your internal thermostat. Studies have shown that our immune cells are able to fight infections better and harder at elevated temperatures. We also know that higher temperatures decrease the ability of pathogens to multiply, slowing the rate of infection.

So although a fever seems bad and scary, when an otherwise healthy person's temperature begins to rise, it is HIGHLY UNLIKELY that it will cause any kind of brain damage, even if a child has a seizure due to rapidly escalating body temperature. The truth is this: The time to be worried about a high fever being

R℞ PRESCRIPTION FROM DR. LOW DOG
Making Sense of the Medication for Munchkins

It's perfectly reasonable to use OTC pain-relief medications in acute situations. They make your child more comfortable and help keep the fever manageable. I generally recommend giving a dose in the late afternoon or early evening, when fever and discomfort generally worsen. When giving pain and fever medicines to children, remember the following:

Acetaminophen (Tylenol) is approved for children 2 months and older.
Ibuprofen (Motrin or Advil) is approved for children 6 months and older.

Aspirin should not be given to children under the age of 18 because of the risk of a dangerous and possibly fatal illness called Reye's syndrome.

---

harmful is when it is NOT due to infection. A heatstroke, when the body is exposed to high environmental temperatures with inadequate fluid intake, is dangerous and definitely can cause brain and organ damage because the heat is due to external causes and is not being regulated by the body's internal thermostat.

☎ Call Your Health Care Provider
- When an otherwise healthy child or adult has a fever of 103°F or higher but is eating and drinking
- When any fever lasts longer than three days

Managing Fever

It's important to remember that a fever is helping the body fight off an infection. You want to make the person comfortable, but not eliminate the fever completely. If a child is able to play or an adult can still do daily activities, there is no reason to do anything more than provide support with healthy broths, herbal teas, and plenty of liquids. However, fevers of 103°F or higher tend to make both kids and adults feel miserable, so using a pain and fever reliever makes sense. If the fever is accompanied by sore throat, diarrhea, or vomiting, follow the recommendations made in those sections. Remember: YOU ARE NOT TREATING THE FEVER, you are supporting the body in defending against whatever is CAUSING the fever.

One of the most important things you can do when fighting an infection is rest. Sleep when you can, and drink plenty of fluids while awake. Although many clinicians recommend "tepid"

Fever Tea

1 teaspoon chamomile flowers
1 teaspoon elder flowers
1 teaspoon lemon balm (may use peppermint in those over 5 years of age)
1 teaspoon maple syrup or honey
2 cups water

Pour 2 cups of near-boiling water over the herbs and let the mixture steep for 5 minutes. Strain. You can add 1 teaspoon of maple syrup for a child under the age of 12 months, or honey for anyone older.

How to Use: For babies 3 to 6 months, give 2 teaspoons every hour or two. For children 6 to 12 months old, give 1 to 2 tablespoons every hour or two. Older children and adults should drink freely.

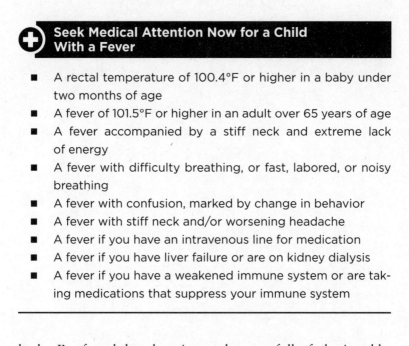

Seek Medical Attention Now for a Child With a Fever

- A rectal temperature of 100.4°F or higher in a baby under two months of age
- A fever of 101.5°F or higher in an adult over 65 years of age
- A fever accompanied by a stiff neck and extreme lack of energy
- A fever with difficulty breathing, or fast, labored, or noisy breathing
- A fever with confusion, marked by change in behavior
- A fever with stiff neck and/or worsening headache
- A fever if you have an intravenous line for medication
- A fever if you have liver failure or are on kidney dialysis
- A fever if you have a weakened immune system or are taking medications that suppress your immune system

---

baths, I've found that these just make most folks feel miserable. If you're feeling cold, sitting in a tepid bath makes you shiver, driving your fever up. I find most people do better if they dress lightly and comfortably, and put on a blanket when chilled and remove it when feeling hot.

Adults and children should make sure to take in plenty of liquids, soups, and broths to provide nourishment and calories, as well as fluid. Breast-fed babies should be encouraged to nurse frequently. Formula-fed babies should be offered their bottle on a regular schedule with water or diluted juice offered in between feedings. The recipe for Fever Tea, opposite, has herbs that help the body fight viral infections. It is calming and relaxing and can help the body manage fever. It is safe for all.

Chapter 3

Caring for the Respiratory System

The respiratory system is made up of the organs and tissues that are involved in breathing, essentially the nasal and sinus cavities, mouth, throat, and lungs. For the purposes of this book, I'm going to focus primarily on the upper respiratory tract, as it is the site of many common problems that are highly amenable to home treatment. I have chosen not to include more serious problems such as asthma, pneumonia, or influenza, as I believe these are best cared for in partnership with your health care provider.

The Defense Team

The upper respiratory system is exquisitely designed to take in air, warm and moisten it, and then move it down through the trachea and into the lungs. But with all this movement of air, it also makes it the most vulnerable interface between our external environment and our inner body. It's estimated that we inhale thousands of organisms every single day. Organisms, such as viruses and bacteria, can easily gain access to our respiratory tract through the inhalation of airborne droplets or by picking up viruses from the hands and then transferring them to the mouth or nose. If our defense system is functioning optimally, the organisms stay localized in our nose, sinuses, and throat. If they invade the lungs, the infection can become far more dangerous.

The good news is that the respiratory tract was built for defense. The hairs in the nose act like a filter to trap larger particles like hair, while the mucosal membrane acts like flypaper, trapping smaller particles, such as viruses, bacteria, and pollen. We may sneeze these out, or remove them by blowing our nose or more commonly by swallowing them. Our stomach acid quickly and thoroughly destroys these microbes. This is why people who are on proton pump inhibitors, drugs that shut off stomach acid, have been found to have an increased risk of pneumonia. As an aside, herbs with a bitter taste enhance the production of stomach acid and other digestive enzymes, which may explain why herbalists have long considered them to be an integral part of maintaining immune health. (See more on both of these topics in Chapter 5.)

For those that sneak past the first line of defense, the adenoids and tonsils—lymph organs in the back of the throat—are ready to sound the alarm and mobilize defender cells. Many baby boomers had their tonsils and adenoids removed as children in the belief that it would reduce childhood ear, nose, and throat infections. However, the Infectious Disease Society of America and American Academy of Pediatrics have concluded removing them does no or little good for reducing the vast majority of these infections and recommend that these tissues only be considered for removal in those who experience extreme and frequent strep throat infections that cannot otherwise be treated with medication.

Finally, the upper respiratory tract is home to many friendly bacteria that help us fight off infection. They do so by competing for binding sites so that harmful microbes have no place to attach, and by producing substances called bacterio-cins, which kill bacteria. One must always keep in mind that most antibiotics destroy the healthy microflora in the back of the throat, making it easy to contract a bacterial infection such as strep throat within months of taking them. I cannot stress enough the need to reserve the use of antibiotics for those infections that really require them, and to include fermented and probiotic rich foods in the diet. Always take a probiotic supplement if you are treated with an antibiotic (see Chapter 2).

You can take additional steps to keep your upper respiratory tract functioning optimally.

Keep Things Moist

Many viruses, especially those that cause colds and influenza, thrive in low humidity, making the nasal passages drier and the mucosal membranes less able to trap them. One of the most helpful things you can do to maintain upper respiratory health is to keep your nasal passages moist. Having lived in the American Southwest most of my life, I have long recommended using a humidifier, but make sure to keep it clean. Dirty reservoirs and filters can quickly breed bacteria and mold—nasty stuff you don't want dispersed into the air you're breathing! You can clean your humidifier with hydrogen peroxide every couple of days and change the filter regularly. I add three to five drops of lavender, rosemary, eucalyptus, or peppermint oil to the water reservoir of my humidifier. The essential oil helps reduce the growth of bacteria and mold, and it makes the air smell nice.

If you should get a stuffy nose, rinsing your nose with a buffered saline solution will reduce nasal swelling, thin the mucus, and make it easier to clear. For babies or infants, most of the distress of a stuffy nose is nasal obstruction, so using saline irrigation and physically removing the mucus can make it easier for them to breathe, nurse, and sleep. Everyone should know how to make a simple saline solution that young and old alike can use to relieve nasal congestion due to colds, seasonal allergies, and dust.

Saline Solution

¼ teaspoon noniodized kosher salt
⅛ teaspoon baking soda
1 cup (8 ounces) boiled or distilled water
Clean jar for solution

Mix water with salt and baking soda. Stir well until salt and soda have dissolved. This solution can be stored up to 24 hours.

Note: Baking soda is a buffering agent that makes the saltwater less irritating to your nose. If you don't have baking soda, just omit from the recipe. I recommend noniodized kosher salt because iodine can be potentially allergenic, and sea salt can contain algae and other contaminants. Always use boiled or distilled water when making your saline solution.

Saline Irrigation for Babies and Young Children

Place your baby on a large bath towel and lay her on her back with her head and shoulders slightly elevated. Make sure your saline solution is room temperature and that you have a clean jar/cup of plain room-temperature water where you can easily access it. Take the bulb syringe, squeeze slightly, and place the tip into the saline solution and release, allowing a small amount of solution to enter into the syringe. Gently put two drops of saline solution in each nostril and then squeeze out any liquid into the cup with tap water. Wait for 30 to 60 seconds. Squeeze the bulb syringe in the palm of your hand and then gently place the tip into the nostril opening, making a tight seal and then release the bulb, sucking up the mucus with the vacuum created. Remove the syringe and squeeze the contents into the cup of tap water. Now take the bulb syringe, squeeze it in the palm of your hand, and insert into the other nostril. Release the bulb and suck out the mucus. Remove the syringe and empty the contents into the cup of tap water. Repeat the entire process one more time. To avoid irritation, limit to two times a day, particularly once before bed, for three to four days. Make sure to thoroughly clean the bulb syringe with warm soapy water and rinse well after each use.

Saline Irrigation for Older Kids and Adults

The most complete way to flush the nose of bacteria-filled mucus, pollen, and dust is with saline solution and a neti pot. Neti pots have been used to perform nasal irrigation in India since ancient times and are now widely recommended by physicians. Typically made of glass or ceramic and looking like a teapot, they can be purchased at many pharmacies, health food stores, and online retailers, and come with instructions for use. Most of my patients have found that using a neti pot dramatically reduces their need for cold and/or allergy medications.

Fill the neti pot with room-temperature saline solution. Standing with your head over the sink, tilt your head about 45 degrees and insert the spout into your top nostril. The solution will flow through your nasal passage and drain out the other nostril. If it drains down your throat, just spit it out. Gently blow your nose to get rid of any remaining solution, refill the neti pot, and repeat in the other nostril. Do this once a day while you have symptoms. If you suffer from seasonal allergies, do this every day for 10 to 14 days and then three times a week. Thoroughly clean the neti pot with warm soapy water after each use.

A Multivitamin a Day Keeps the Doctor Away

I suggest most people consider taking a multivitamin that provides a daily dose of 1,000 IU vitamin D_3, 15 to 20 milligrams zinc, and a minimum of 100 milligrams vitamin C, along with other important vitamins and minerals. Vitamin C and zinc can give your body an edge against colds, while a growing body of evidence suggests that being vitamin D deficient puts you at increased risk for upper respiratory infections. There's even more evidence that the vast majority of Americans are vitamin D deficient. There is no harm in taking 1,000 to 2,000 IU of vitamin D_3 a day. The Institute of Medicine has set the safe level for vitamin D at 4,000 IU a day for those 9 years and older and 2,500 IU a day for children 12 months and older.

Yogurt, Garlic, and More

Of course, don't let taking a multivitamin be an excuse for not eating plenty of vegetables and fruits—they provide a much broader array of nutrients than can ever be found in a vitamin pill! And while you're at it, load up on garlic and onions, both of which have been shown to give your immune system a boost! One study found that eating a cup of probiotic-rich yogurt daily lowered the risk of getting a cold. As mentioned previously, it's important to maintain healthy levels of friendly microbes.

The upper respiratory system does an amazing job protecting us from harm, as well as allowing us to experience all the tastes and smells of our world. I have chosen to cover some of the most common complaints that I've seen over and over again in my practice. Colds, coughs, ear infections, sore throats, allergies, and cold sores can be easily managed at home using gentle and effective remedies. Although I have chosen not to discuss asthma or more severe respiratory infections, you will find that many of the recommendations in the following sections can be helpful for these, as well.

► Cold Comfort: Colds, Sniffles, and Stuffy Noses

Get ready to be hit by at least one cold, maybe more, this year. Consider: The average adult gets two to four colds a year. And if you've got kids, stock up on tissue and chicken soup. Children typically come down with more than twice the colds that adults do.

More than 200 viruses, and a small number of bacteria, are responsible for what is medically known as acute nasopharyngitis (inflammation of the nose and throat) or acute upper respiratory tract infections (URIs). In everyday language, we call these "common colds." URIs are more common during the fall and winter months, as the air becomes drier and humidity levels fall. Central heat, furnaces, and woodstoves make the air even drier inside your home and office, leading to dry, irritated nasal passages. Small cracks develop in this delicate but highly protective barrier tissue lining your nose, sinuses, and throat. Your first line of defense is thus breached, allowing viruses and bacteria to gain a foothold. When the weather is cold, we also tend to stay inside more, increasing our contact with one another and making it easier to transmit viruses.

Children have an average of four to eight URIs a year, with the highest number occurring in children under the age of two. This is often the result of being in day care, school, or at home with other little kids, sharing toys, crayons, books, and other items and not washing their hands regularly. URIs in young children are generally more troubling than in teens and adults, causing fever, irritability, nasal congestion, and often ear pain and/or infection. Other than trying to reduce exposure for babies under the age of three months, you can't do much to prevent getting colds. And, as I discussed in the previous chapter on infections, before you start thinking that there's something wrong with your child, science has shown that these infections in childhood are important for training the immune system to discern what is and is not harmful.

Those stuffy noses, nighttime coughing, and general irritability can be rough on both kids and parents. Children often cannot go to day care or school, which means someone has to stay home to take care of them. Although not a hardship in some families, the loss of pay for others can be devastating. All of these problems and frustrations drive many parents to the urgent care for antibiotics, which are not effective, and/or to the pharmacy for over-the-counter (OTC) cough and cold medicines. But read the labels: You'll find that virtually all of these products instruct you to talk to your physician before giving to a child aged four to six, and not to use in any child under the age of four.

These scary but important warnings are the result of a petition sent to the Food and Drug Administration (FDA) in 2007 by a group of physicians who wanted parents to know that these cold medications were neither effective nor safe in young children, particularly if the recommended dose was exceeded. The FDA didn't ban these medications but recommended that kids under age four not take them. After the FDA's guidance was published, the number of emergency room visits for side effects due to these medications decreased by 50 percent. Still, countless parents were at a loss for what they should do to help their children feel better.

In the aftermath of the FDA's recommendations, I was invited to speak about treating kids with URIs on numerous radio and television shows. What's more, I was flooded with emails and

R̲X̲ | PRESCRIPTION FROM DR. LOW DOG

Is It Allergies?

Seasonal allergies, also known as allergic rhinitis or hay fever, are an all-too-common problem for many of us. The classic symptoms of sneezing, watery eyes, stuffy nose, and itchy nose and throat can sometimes be confused with URIs; however, allergies do not cause the low-grade fever that usually accompanies a cold. See the section on Seasonal Allergies (pages 114–118) for more information on how you can manage at home.

phone calls from colleagues and parents who wanted to know about the safety of some of the "alternative" remedies being recommended, such as echinacea, elderberry, zinc, and vitamin C. Could a two-year-old take echinacea, and if so, how much? What did I recommend for a persistent cough?

I'd never realized that so many people relied so heavily upon these OTC products. With the exception of acetaminophen (Tylenol) or ibuprofen (Motrin, Advil) for pain or fever, I'd never used any of these cold products in my kids, nor recommended them for patients. For the vast majority of children and adults, simple home remedies, hydration, rest, and tender loving care (TLC) are all that is needed.

Fast Relief With Aromatherapy

Aromatic plants and their oils have long been used for their medicinal, cleansing, and mood-enhancing effects. The therapeutic use of these aromatic oils is called aromatherapy.

- *Aromatherapy steam.* Fill a large saucepan with water and bring to a boil on the stove. Remove it from the heat and place it on a heat-safe surface. Let it cool for a couple of minutes, and then add 3 to 5 drops of essential oil. Tent your head with a large bath towel over the pan, close your eyes, and breathe in slowly for about 5 to 10 minutes. Keep your face 15 to 18 inches above the pan to prevent burning your skin.

- *Aromatherapy compress.* Dampen a washcloth with very warm (not hot) water. Add 3 drops essential oil. Lie down, close your eyes, and drape the warm washcloth over your face for 3 to 5 minutes. The heat and moisture will help reduce nasal swelling and ease a sinus headache. Repeat as needed.

My favorite herbal essential oils to use in any method of aromatherapy treatment for colds and stuffy noses are:

- *Eucalyptus.* This all-time classic is an antiviral that soothes the respiratory system and clears the nose.
- *Oregano.* If your head feels like the overstuffed chair in your living room, this antiviral and antioxidant oil helps knock out low-grade sinus infections.
- *Peppermint.* This essential oil is simply the best if your stuffy nose is giving you a headache.
- *Rosemary.* Another antiviral, rosemary is a powerful antiseptic and decongestant. Some say you shouldn't use rosemary oil for aromatherapy if you're pregnant because it might cause uterine contractions. I find that hard to believe, but it might be better to opt for one of the others mentioned here.

Zinc Lozenges

Studies have shown that zinc lozenges can reduce the severity and shorten the duration of a cold. I recommend lozenges containing 5 to 10 milligrams of elemental zinc, as those with higher levels tend to upset the stomach and leave a metallic taste in your mouth. You can safely take up to 80 milligrams a day for

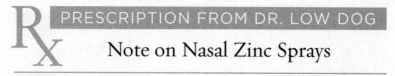

PRESCRIPTION FROM DR. LOW DOG
Note on Nasal Zinc Sprays

Alert: Should you try zinc nasal sprays? Probably not—for two reasons. First, using zinc nasal sprays has been rumored to destroy your sense of smell, although the evidence is not conclusive. Second, there isn't any concrete evidence that putting zinc in your nose is any better than taking it orally. Until we know more about their effectiveness, I would avoid using zinc nasal sprays.

five days, but you shouldn't take more than 20 to 30 milligrams a day of zinc long-term without also taking 0.5 to 1.0 milligram a day of copper (zinc depletes copper). The most absorbable forms are zinc glycinate and zinc gluconate.

Herbal Teas

On those nights when I feel like I'm "coming down with a cold," I turn to ginger, one of my favorite herbal teas. Ginger has antiviral and anti-inflammatory activity, helping to destroy viruses that cause upper respiratory infections, shrinking nasal swelling, and soothing a sore throat. This popular spice will warm you

PRESCRIPTION FROM DR. LOW DOG
Honey to the Rescue

Got a cold? This is a great time to pull out the medicinal honeys you've made. Garlic honey is awesome for a cold, and if you've got a sore throat or cough, consider sage or thyme! (See the medicinal honey recipes in "The Eighteen Essentials.")

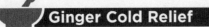

Ginger Cold Relief

1 inch fresh ginger rhizome (root) cut into slices OR $\frac{1}{2}$ teaspoon
   dried ginger
1 teaspoon honey
1 teaspoon lemon juice
$1\frac{1}{2}$ cups (12 ounces) water

Put water into a saucepan, add ginger, and gently bring to a
boil. Cover and simmer on very low heat for 15 to 20 minutes.
Strain and add honey and lemon juice.

How to Use: Teens and adults should drink 1 to 3 times a day.
Children under the age of 12 months can drink $\frac{1}{4}$ to $\frac{1}{2}$ cup, 1 to
3 times a day, depending on age.

*Awesome cold reliever. If you want an extra anti-inflammatory,
antiviral boost, you can add $\frac{1}{2}$ teaspoon licorice root when
cooking your ginger. Licorice is particularly helpful for soothing
a bad sore throat. Except for those with high blood pressure,
adding this amount of licorice is perfectly fine for 2 to 3 days.*

---

from your fingers to your toes, making it great for those times
when you feel like you've taken a chill. I prefer fresh ginger for
colds and coughs, but you can use dried if that's what you've
got around the house and don't feel like running to the grocery
store. The above remedy is delicious, easy to make, and safe and
effective for anyone over the age of two.

Echinacea

I've had a long and enduring relationship with echinacea, also
known as purple coneflower. I've treated at least a thousand
people with the tea or tincture over the years and have not found

it wanting. I've taken it myself and given it to my children on countless occasions. Called *icahpehu* in Lakota for "strike-down stem," the roots of *Echinacea angustifolia* and *E. purpurea* were used extensively by Native Americans to treat tonsillitis, coughs, toothaches, snakebites, and skin diseases. Early physicians in the United States highly valued it and used it widely, but it fell out of favor with the discovery of penicillin and other antibiotics. Modern studies show that it revs up the immune system, allowing the body to respond more rapidly and efficiently to eliminate

Echinacea Apricot Tincture

60 grams *E. purpurea* dried root, ground or chopped
300 milliliters brandy (80 to 100 proof)
10 unsulfured dried apricots, sliced
1 tablespoon honey (optional)

Grind echinacea to a coarse powder and put in a large wide-mouthed canning jar. Add brandy, honey, and apricots. Stir well and cover with a lid. If more liquid is needed, add another 60 milliliters brandy. Shake daily and let sit for 2 to 4 weeks. Strain and pour into a dark colored bottle. Label and store in a dark, cool place.

How to Use: Teens and adults: Take 1 teaspoon of the tincture every 3 to 4 hours if you feel like you're coming down with a cold or sore throat. Do this for the first 48 hours, and chances are you might avoid getting sick all together!

Children 12 and under: Take $\frac{1}{4}$ to $\frac{1}{2}$ teaspoon every 3 to 4 hours, depending upon age. This tincture has a small amount of honey, so isn't suitable for children under one year of age. (I generally give children echinacea glycerite, as it doesn't contain any alcohol and they generally prefer the taste.)

viral and bacterial infections. These effects are most pronounced the first 72 hours of taking the herb.

You can purchase echinacea tincture online or at health food stores, but it's cheaper to make your own. See the basic recipe in "The Eighteen Essentials," pages 282–283, or try the delicious and highly effective Echinacea Apricot Tincture recipe above. I usually make a big batch and give some away as gifts to friends and family in early autumn, so that everyone is set for cold and flu season.

Note: Echinacea is a member of the Aster family, and someone might have an allergic reaction to it on rare occasions. In all my years of practice, I have actually only *seen* it once in a five-year-old who had a strong history of asthma and eczema. Within ten minutes after taking a dose of echinacea glycerite, he developed a small red itchy ring around his mouth, clearly an allergic reaction. So, although it's rare, far more rare than allergies to peanuts, it can happen, especially in those who have a severe allergy to the daisy family.

Kiara's Cherry-Echinacea Glycerite

60 grams *E. purpurea* root, ground or chopped
240 milliliters kosher vegetable glycerin
60 milliliters dark cherry juice OR
60 milliliters distilled water + 20 drops natural cherry flavoring

In a large saucepan, put vegetable glycerine and cherry juice OR distilled water and stir until blended on very low heat. Add echinacea, and on the lowest setting, gently heat, covered for 10 minutes. Remove from heat and let steep for 10 minutes. Without straining, pour into a widemouthed canning jar. If you used distilled water, you can add the natural cherry flavoring at this time. Cover with a lid. Let it sit for 2 to 4 weeks.

If you need to add more liquid, add 40 milliliters vegetable glycerin and 20 milliliters water or dark cherry juice. When ready, remove the lid and put the jar into a saucepan that contains 1 to 2 inches of water. Bring water to a low boil and gently stir the mixture in the jar until it becomes slightly runny. Using a hot pad or mitt, carefully remove the jar and pour the liquid through a cheesecloth-lined strainer into a bowl. Then using a funnel, pour the liquid into a clean, dark-colored bottle and label. This glycerite will stay good for roughly 2 years and is suitable for all ages.

How to Use: Children for up to 5 days:

15 to 25 pounds: $1/2$ teaspoon every 2 to 3 hours
25 to 50 pounds: $3/4$ teaspoon every 2 to 3 hours
50 to 75 pounds: 1 teaspoon every 2 to 3 hours
75 to 100 pounds: $1 1/2$ teaspoons every 2 to 3 hours

This remedy was my daughter Kiara's favorite growing up. On those days when she'd come home with sniffles and a scratchy throat, she'd ask for her "etch-in-a-chea" and happily take a teaspoonful without fuss. I figured being a kid was hard enough without having to take a yucky medicine when you're feeling bad. Though not as "strong" as a tincture made with alcohol, vegetable glycerin is the preferred solvent for children, in my opinion. You simply give them a little bit more to make up the difference.

|||||||||||||||||||||||||||||||||||||||||||||||||||||||||||||||||||||||||||||||||||||||||||||||||||||||

☎ Call Your Health Care Provider

- When a fever reaches 103°F or higher or when ANY fever lasts longer than three days in an otherwise healthy child or adult who is eating, drinking, and not having difficulty breathing

|||||||||||||||||||||||||||||||||||||||||||||||||||||||||||||||||||||||||||||||||||||||||||||||||||||||

R_X PRESCRIPTION FROM DR. LOW DOG

Is It Asthma?

Approximately 30 percent of children with asthma are symptomatic by the time they are one year of age, and 80 to 90 percent will have had symptoms by the time they are five years old. Acute wheezing can occur after an exposure to aspirin, cold air, tobacco smoke, or an allergen. When children have a URI, symptoms are often more gradual with increased coughing and wheezing, particularly at night, developing after a few days. If you notice your child has repeated episodes of coughing and wheezing, especially when she has a cold, or after exercising or being exposed to certain foods or chemicals, you should definitely have your child evaluated for asthma. If your child has a URI, the main thing to be on the lookout for is any kind of respiratory distress: difficulty breathing, flaring nostrils, or prolonged exhalation. If any of these are present, take your child immediately to the emergency room or urgent care.

 Seek Medical Attention Now for Cold Symptoms

- When there is shortness of breath, breathing difficulty, nasal flaring, or any wheezing
- When a baby under two months of age has a fever of 100.4°F or higher
- When an infant who has had a mild URI for a couple of days suddenly spikes a temperature over 102°F and has difficulty breathing (this may indicate pneumonia)
- When any child, teen, or adult with a mild URI suddenly develops a shaking chill followed by a rapid rise in temperature and hacking cough (this is a typical presentation for pneumonia in this age group)

◆ Ease a Cough

Whether it wakes you up at night, kicks in the minute you start talking on the phone, or is just that annoying tickle in the back of your throat—we've all experienced coughing. Coughs let you know that something's wrong: that too much mucous, stomach acid, or smoke has irritated nerves in the passages leading to your lungs. Coughing is your body's way of trying to get rid of the irritant. Acute coughs last for less than three weeks and are most commonly caused by upper respiratory infections and seasonal allergies. A cough is considered "chronic" if it lasts for more than eight weeks. Any chronic cough should be evaluated by a health professional, though the most common causes are postnasal drip, asthma, and gastroesophageal reflux disease (GERD). (See Chapter 5 for more information on this last condition.) Persistent coughing drives people crazy, explaining why it is the most common reason people see their primary care provider.

||||||||||||||||||||||||||||||||||||||||||||||||||||||||||||||||||||||||||||||||||||||||||||||||||||||||||

☎ Call Your Health Care Provider
■　If your cough doesn't go away in eight weeks

||||||||||||||||||||||||||||||||||||||||||||||||||||||||||||||||||||||||||||||||||||||||||||||||||||||||||

Herbal Cough Relievers
Herbs that relieve coughs are called "antitussives." Some of the most commonly used are marshmallow root and leaf, mullein leaf and flowers, mallow leaf and flowers, slippery elm, and plantain. These herbs are rich in mucopolysaccharides, compounds that form a gel when they come into contact with water. Taken as a tea, this gelatinous material coats and soothes by preventing activation of the irritant receptors that line the

throat. Remember, if you can soothe the irritation, you can reduce the cough.

I've included some of my favorite cough remedies that I've used over the past three decades. They range from marshmallow tea, slippery elm lozenges, and thyme syrup to more complex formulations I've developed for those who needed stronger medicine.

Thyme Cough Syrup

4 tablespoons fresh thyme
1 teaspoon lemon juice
1 cup water
$1/4$ cup honey, preferably raw and local OR
$1/4$ cup maple syrup if using for a child under 12 months of age

Pour near-boiling water over thyme and steep, covered, for 15 minutes. Strain. Add honey and lemon juice. Refrigerate for up to 1 week. For children 12 months and older: Give 1 to 2 teaspoons every 2 to 3 hours, as needed. Teens and adults can take 1 to 2 tablespoons every 2 to 3 hours, as needed.

For children under the age of 12 months, substitute maple syrup for the honey and give $1/2$ teaspoon every 2 to 3 hours, as needed. Maple syrup comes from inside the maple tree and is then boiled at high heat, making the risk of infant botulism from maple syrup virtually nonexistent, according to the Centers for Disease Control.

Thyme is definitely my go-to acute cough syrup because it works quickly, tastes great, is very safe, and costs so little to make. The common garden thyme is one of our most trusted and respected herbs for relieving coughs and congestion. In fact, the German health authorities endorse the use of thyme for treating acute and chronic bronchitis, whooping cough, and URIs. The essential oil fraction of the herb—the compounds that give thyme its aroma—makes the mucus thinner and easier to expectorate or cough up, and acts as an antiseptic and antibacterial in the lungs. To get the most benefit from thyme, use the fresh herb, which you should be able to find throughout the year in the produce section of most grocery stores.

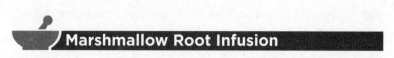
Marshmallow Root Infusion

1 heaping teaspoon marshmallow root, dried and chopped
1 cup purified water

Put the chopped marshmallow root into a mug and add room-temperature water. Cover and let it sit for 2 to 3 hours. Strain the liquid through a tea strainer.

How to Use: Drink $1/2$ cup 2 to 3 times a day.

Few herbs are more healing for the throat, esophagus, and stomach than marshmallow leaves or root. The Romans ate marshmallow leaves in their soups and stews, while physicians in the United Kingdom made a hard candy from the juiced roots, egg whites, and sugar to soothe children's sore throats. Marshmallows bought in a grocery store today are a pale shadow of this original. Marshmallow contains mucilage, which protects and eases irritated mucosal membranes. The herb is completely safe and gentle enough for any age.

Grindelia Compound Tincture

This is a formula I've used for years for acute and chronic coughs (recipe, pages 283–284). It opens up the chest, dilating the bronchioles, making it easier to breathe. The combination of herbs helps shrink nasal passages, reducing postnasal drip; soothes an irritated throat; helps the body fight off viral infections; and thins sputum, making it easier to expectorate. I keep the tincture on hand at all times so that I can make up the syrup whenever needed.

Slippery Elm

Slippery elm bark has been used to soothe throat irritation for centuries. The FDA still recognizes slippery elm bark as a safe and effective oral demulcent (tissue soother). You can buy slippery elm lozenges at the store, make your own (see the recipe below), or drink it as tea. Since the herbal component here is tree bark, make the tea as a decoction. Slippery elm is safe for all ages.

Slippery Elm Lozenges

The inner bark of the North American elm tree has been used for many centuries to soothe sore throats or ease heartburn. In fact, the FDA has declared that slippery elm is a safe and effective oral demulcent, meaning that it relieves inflammation and irritation.

Powdered slippery elm bark is perfectly safe for young and old. It can be prepared as a tea, taken as gruel, or easily made into throat lozenges. I like lozenges because you can be creative with them. I've made batches with natural cherry flavoring, essential oils, maple syrup, and fruit juice. My kids loved to help me make them.

$1/2$ cup slippery elm bark powder
$1/8$ teaspoon cinnamon powder or pumpkin pie spice (optional)
$1/3$ cup honey or maple syrup

Put the slippery elm powder and cinnamon or pumpkin pie spice into the mixing bowl and stir to blend. Then make a little well in the middle and add the honey or maple syrup. Mix well. It should have a consistency like Play-Doh. You can add more slippery elm powder or more maple syrup or honey, as needed.

Next, coat your hands with a little slippery elm powder, and then roll small pieces of the dough into marble-size balls. The slippery elm powder keeps the dough from sticking to your hands. The lozenges will stay fresh for months in an airtight container.

If you want to get fancy, sprinkle slippery elm powder on a sheet of waxed paper. Then use a rolling pin until the dough is about $\frac{1}{4}$ inch thick. Use a small candy cutter or the cap from a small bottle to make your lozenges. Sprinkle with a little extra slippery elm powder and store in an airtight container.

How to Use: Suck on a lozenge every 1 to 3 hours for a sore throat. Slippery elm lozenges can be used to ease a sore throat, no matter the cause. Here are three variations:

Option 1: If you've made any medicinal honeys, like sage or thyme, use these instead of plain honey to increase the antibacterial and throat-soothing effects.

Option 2: Use 2 tablespoons honey and 2 tablespoons dark cherry concentrate, and leave out the cinnamon or pumpkin pie spice. Make exactly the same way as the original recipe.

Option 3: Make the original recipe but leave out the cinnamon/ pumpkin pie spice and add 4 to 5 drops essential oil for flavor and additional antiseptic activity. Some good choices include peppermint or clove bud oil.

R̶X PRESCRIPTION FROM DR. LOW DOG
Honey for Cough

Winnie the Pooh was definitely on to something with his love of honey! Studies have shown that honey is highly effective for relieving nighttime coughing in children over the age of one. As a matter of fact, researchers found that honey is as effective as dextromethorphan, a common cough suppressant, and more effective than diphenhydramine, a common antihistamine. Different types of honey have been used in this research, and all of them worked! The dose was 1 to 2 teaspoons before bed, and both children and their parents were able to get a good night's sleep! You can do this one even better, however, by using sage or thyme medicinal honey (see recipes in Chapter 9).

Seek Immediate Medical Attention if You Have a Cough With:

- Bloody sputum
- Shortness of breath, difficulty breathing
- Chest pain

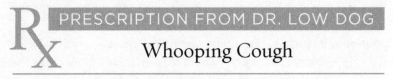

R℞ PRESCRIPTION FROM DR. LOW DOG

Whooping Cough

Pertussis is a bacterial infection that causes inflammation of the lungs and airways. The name "whooping cough" comes from the sound people make gasping for air after a pertussis coughing fit. We are seeing a rise in whooping cough in the United States because a growing number of parents are not immunizing their children, and the protection provided from the newer acellular vaccinations, although safer, wears off more quickly. That means older siblings and adults may spread the infection without knowing it. In fact, up to 20 percent of people with coughs lasting more than two weeks have pertussis! Antibiotics shorten duration of the cough if caught early. Use steam or humidifiers to keep airways open and moist, remove all dairy products (other than formula), use vitamin C, Thyme Cough Syrup, and Grindelia Compound if two years or older.

◗ Ear Infections

Two scenarios: First, you notice your 15-month-old is rubbing his ear. He's fussy, too, with a runny nose, and a temperature of 101°F. Otherwise, he seems fine. Should you take him to the doctor? It probably isn't necessary.

Second scenario: He's pulling on his ear and crying. You're having trouble soothing him. He's not playing, and his fever's been hovering around 103°F for two days. Should you take him to the doctor? It's probably a good idea.

The difference in these two cases is the severity of the pain and the strength and duration of the fever. The decision to seek medical attention ultimately comes down to your comfort level for treating your child at home. I've often encouraged parents to "become their own pediatrician"—a suggestion that starts with purchasing and learning how to use a basic otoscope for examining their children's ears. Ask your health care provider to teach you how if you have young children. This diagnostic device comes in handy; knowing how to use it can help cut down on unnecessary office visits, and also gives you the confidence to know when to seek medical attention.

But remember to always trust your intuition. It is always better to err on the side of caution! It is NEVER wrong to talk to your doctor or other trusted clinician if you're unsure about whether something can be managed at home.

Some basic ear anatomy: There is a tiny tube called the Eustachian tube that runs from the middle ear to the throat. Every time you swallow, this tube adjusts the pressure in your ear and drains the accumulating fluids; this is the reason your ears "pop" when changing elevation and why it can be painful to fly when your nose is all stuffed up.

When you have a cold, your ears accumulate fluid just like your nose, but if the Eustachian tube becomes blocked, the ear cannot drain, and fluids becomes trapped. You feel pressure and don't hear as well. In infants and young children, the Eustachian tube is shorter and more horizontal than in adolescents and adults, making it harder to drain and easier for bacteria from the nose and throat to reach the ear. (This change in tube anatomy is why children often outgrow ear troubles.) When a child gets an upper respiratory infection, inflammation causes the Eustachian tube to swell shut and trap the fluid, and possibly bacteria, in the middle ear.

The first scenario described previously is called otitis media with effusion (OME). This is the medical term for a buildup of fluid in the middle ear. It is most often caused by viral upper respiratory infections, allergies, or exposure to irritants like cigarette smoke. The second scenario describes another type of childhood ear infection called acute otitis media (AOM). This is the medical term for the rapid onset of inflammation in the middle ear, which usually causes pain, redness of the eardrum, and fever. A parent can distinguish between these two with a home otoscope.

There are certain signs that suggest an ear infection, such as: The ear canal is red, swollen, or filled with pus; the eardrum is red and bulging; or there is a hole in the eardrum. An otoscope also helps you see if there is excessive earwax or if the child has put a foreign object, such as a bead, into the ear canal. Older children pull on the affected ear, and infants become very irritable. Severe AOM occurs when there is moderate to severe ear pain and a fever of 102.2°F or higher.

Many physicians will prescribe an antibiotic for severe AOM. If you decide to give your child the antibiotic, make sure you give it for the full amount of time on the label. Stopping the treatment midcourse can lead to the development of resistant strains of bacteria and make the next infection more difficult to treat. And any time your child takes antibiotics, make sure to supplement

R̲X PRESCRIPTION FROM DR. LOW DOG
OTC Painkillers and Kids

Although some parents are reluctant to use over-the-counter pain relievers, I think they are perfectly fine for short-term use (two to four days). When the pain is under control, children are more likely to eat, drink, and sleep, all of which help them heal. Look for acetaminophen or ibuprofen, without any other ingredients added. Acetaminophen is best for children under six months of age; otherwise, I recommend ibuprofen. Liquids and chewable forms are available, depending upon the age of your child. Follow the directions based upon your child's age and/or weight.

with probiotics both during treatment and for at least six to eight weeks afterward. The strains that have the best evidence in adults and children are *Saccharomyces boulardii* and *Lactobacillus* GG. The latter is available in forms specifically for young infants.

The American Academy of Pediatrics (AAP) now recommends giving parents the option of waiting 48 to 72 hours to see if symptoms resolve on their own before using an antibiotic. This is because roughly two-thirds of kids with AOM will get better without them. Antibiotics are overprescribed, particularly in children, leading to resistant bacteria and infections that are difficult to treat. The AAP recommends offering over-the-counter pain relievers, such as children's acetaminophen or ibuprofen, and monitoring a child's temperature. Antibiotics are prescribed if a child worsens or fails to improve in two to three days.

Mommy Strategies: Treating an Acute Ear Infection at Home

- *Nasal irrigation.* One of the most important things you can do to prevent and/or treat an ear infection is to keep the nasal passages as clear as possible if there are any signs of a cold or upper respiratory infection. This will help the Eustachian tube stay open, and reduce the number of bacteria in the nose and throat. Follow the saline irrigation instructions on pages 84–86).

- *Immune support.* I remain a fan of echinacea for giving the immune system a boost. Refer to the section on echinacea tinctures and glycerites in the section titled "Cold Comfort," pages 92–95, for dosing and preparation instructions.

- *Zinc and vitamin C.* Because most ear infections are associated with upper respiratory infections, using zinc lozenges for children old enough to suck on them, and giving extra vitamin C (100 milligrams 3 to 4 times a day) will help with both.

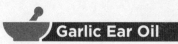

Garlic Ear Oil

2 cloves fresh garlic
Extra virgin olive oil or mullein oil

Chop two cloves of fresh garlic and let sit for 10 minutes. Then put the garlic into the top of a double boiler and add $\frac{1}{4}$ cup olive oil (or your strained mullein oil). Cook over very low heat for 15 minutes. If you don't have a double boiler, you can use a saucepan over very low heat, but stir frequently to prevent scorching the oil. Strain well and let the oil cool completely. Place the liquid in a jar with a tight-fitting lid and use within a week.

How to Use: Lie on side with affected ear facing up. Put 2 to 3 drops into the ear. Gently push and pull the outer ear to work the oil down into the canal. Lie in this position for about 5 minutes. You can use a cotton ball to keep the oil in the ear canal. Repeat 2 to 3 times a day.

Note: Never put cold oil into the ear, as it can cause severe dizziness. And never put hot oil in the ear, as it can burn!

I've used garlic oil many times over the years with great success. However, I've had a handful of occasions in which it actually worsened the ear pain. Once I put a few drops in a child's ears, and he started crying. I gently wiped the ear clean with a cotton swab. When I examined the area, the ear canal was redder than it had been before I used the oil. So a word to the wise: Put 1 drop in the ear the first time you use it. Wait 5 to 10 minutes. If there isn't any problem, proceed as directed.

- *Ear oil.* Ear oils made with mullein flowers, garlic, and/or St. John's wort can help ease ear pain. There are many excellent commercial ear oils on the market, or you can make your own. My favorites are made with garlic (above) or mullein (pages 289–290).

Prevent Recurrent Ear Infections

Seasonal, food, and other allergies are often the primary drivers for recurrent ear infections. Studies have repeatedly shown that formula-fed babies are at higher risk for ear infections, whereas those who are breast-fed for at least 6 months have a lower incidence. If your child has had three or more ear infections in a 12-month period, talk to your health care provider about doing an elimination diet or removing all dairy products from your child's diet for 1 month. If I had a dollar for every child who dramatically improved after being taken off dairy and/or soy, I'd be a wealthy woman today!

Here's something I find interesting: Researchers have shown that pacifier use increases ear infections. The current recommendations are to use them only to help your baby go to sleep once he is six months of age and eliminate them altogether by ten months of age. It's thought that sucking on a pacifier changes the air pressure in the ears and increases the likelihood of the Eustachian tube becoming blocked. If your child is having problems with recurrent ear infections, ditch the pacifier!

Also, keep up with the nasal irrigations, particularly in munchkins with persistent runny noses or stopped-up nasal passages. Buffered saline solution is highly effective, and older children can be taught to use a neti pot or neti-med bottle (see pages 85–86).

Although there is less evidence for probiotics in preventing recurrent ear infections, I still recommend them. Look for a product that contains *Lactobacillus* GG and/or *L. reuteri*.

Relief for Outer Ear Infections

Otitis externa is an infection of the canal that connects the outer ear to the eardrum. Often called "swimmer's ear," this condition can affect anyone who is exposed to wind and rain. Moisture and bacteria are trapped in the outer ear canal, leaving the ears

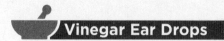
Vinegar Ear Drops

2 tablespoons (1 ounce) water
2 tablespoons (1 ounce) white vinegar
Bottle with eyedropper

Mix the water and vinegar together and put the mixture in a clean container. The acidity in the vinegar will prevent bacteria from growing.

How to Use: Lie on your side with the affected ear facing up. Put 2 to 3 drops directly into the external ear canal and then gently push and pull your ear to work the drops down into the canal to remove any trapped air. Lie in this position for about 5 minutes to ensure that the ear drops do not drain from your ear canal. Leave your ear canal open to dry.

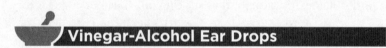
Vinegar-Alcohol Ear Drops

If you are prone to getting swimmer's ear, use this remedy to prevent infection. Don't use this once your ears are hurting, however, because the alcohol will burn.

2 tablespoons (1 ounce) rubbing alcohol
2 tablespoons (1 ounce) white vinegar
Bottle with an eyedropper

Mix the alcohol and vinegar together and put the mixture in a bottle. The alcohol effectively removes the water, while the acidity in the vinegar prevents bacteria from growing. Label the bottle carefully with the words FOR EXTERNAL USE ONLY. You never want to use rubbing alcohol internally.

How to Use: Apply 2 to 3 room-temperature drops in each ear after swimming or showering. Follow directions for use provided under Vinegar Ear Drops.

---

feeling itchy and "plugged up," and they can become red, swollen, and highly sensitive to the touch. The classic sign of an outer ear infection is pain when you tug on the earlobe. The key to preventing these kinds of ear infections is to keep your ears dry. Use a blow-dryer set on low heat to help dry your ears after showering, swimming, or otherwise getting wet.

Although severe cases of *otitis externa* usually require antibiotic ear drops, milder cases can be treated at home with just a little vinegar and water.

||||||||||||||||||||||||||||||||||||||||||||||||||||||||||||||||||||||||||||||||||||||||||||||||||||||||||||||

☎ Consult Your Health Care Provider

- When a baby under three months of age has a fever of 100.4°F or higher
- When ear pain persists or worsens over a 24-hour period in spite of over-the-counter pain relievers
- When a fever is 103°F or higher or any fever lasts longer than three days

||||||||||||||||||||||||||||||||||||||||||||||||||||||||||||||||||||||||||||||||||||||||||||||||||||||||||||||

▶ Sore Throat Soothers

You know the feeling: the sandpapery sensation in your throat, the raspy voice, the painful swallowing. You've got a classic case of sore throat, often indicating the beginning of a cold or the flu. Sore throats, medically known as pharyngitis, are very common, prompting between 16 million and 18 million visits to doctors' offices each year, according to the National Center for Health Statistics.

A sore throat can be the result of bacterial or viral infections or noninfectious causes such as smoking or hay fever. The vast majority of sore throats, however, are hands down due to viral infections, such as the common cold. When the virus invades the mucosal lining of the nose and throat, the tissue becomes swollen and inflamed. Most of the pain and discomfort we experience is actually due to our body's immune response, not the virus.

Viral sore throats are almost always associated with a runny/stuffy nose and a cough. So everything discussed in the section titled "Cold Comfort" holds true for virus-triggered sore throats. Nasal irrigation and steams can be very helpful, as can some of the following timeless remedies.

Sage Gargle

My grandmother used to keep a cup of sage tea containing a pinch of salt by the sink whenever we'd come down with a sore throat. She'd tell us to stop and gargle every time we passed through the kitchen. "The more times, the better," she'd say. We didn't mind because it didn't taste bad and it worked fast.

My grandmother was definitely on to something. A member of the mint family, sage is an old and time-honored remedy for irritation and inflammation of the mouth, throat, and tonsils. But modern science also supports this folk remedy. Two studies have shown that sage, as well as sage in combination with echinacea, was more effective than placebo, and equally as effective as a throat spray containing an antibacterial plus 2 percent lidocaine, a topical anesthetic. The German health authorities recognize sage gargle as a treatment for sore throat.

||||||||||||||||||||||||||||||||||||||||||||||||||||||||||||||||||||||||||||||||||||||||||||||

☎ When to Call Your Health Care Provider

- If you have a persistent sore throat that doesn't clear up within a few days, talk to your health care provider to determine the underlying cause.

||||||||||||||||||||||||||||||||||||||||||||||||||||||||||||||||||||||||||||||||||||||||||||||

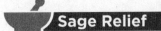

Sage Relief

1 tablespoon fresh sage leaves or 2 teaspoons dried sage
1/4 teaspoon salt
1 cup water

Bring the water to a boil, turn off the heat, add fresh or dried sage, cover, and let steep for 10 minutes. Strain. Pour into a tea mug and add salt. Stir.

How to Use: Gargle every 1 to 2 hours, or as needed, for sore throat. (Don't swallow the sage and salt; just swish and spit.)

This gargle combines really well with echinacea tincture if you're fighting off a cold. It can also be used safely with antibiotic treatment for strep throat. If you've made Sage Medicinal Honey, this would sure be a good time to use it.

Echinacea to the Rescue

I've had my share of sore throats. Some were doozies. I have no idea whether or not some of those sore throats were strep, as I had no health insurance, seldom went to the doctor, and was often out in remote areas without access anyway. What I can tell you is that echinacea worked like a charm every time. Sometimes when I thought it was worse than usual, I'd take barberry tincture with my echinacea. The dose for barberry tincture is 2 to 3 milliliters taken 3 times per day.

Echinacea is one of my favorite herbs for sore throats. It not only helps the body fight off the infection but it also has a mild numbing effect, making it easier to swallow.

For best results, take 5 milliliters echinacea root tincture (see the recipe for Echinacea Tincture in "The Eighteen Essentials," pages 282–283) every 2 to 3 hours at the first sign of a sore throat.

Take this up to 6 times a day for 3 days. The dose can be decreased to 3 times a day for an additional 3 to 4 days, if needed.

Strep Throat

What worries people the most when they get a sore throat is the possibility that it might be strep throat. Only 10 to 20 percent of sore throats are due to streptococcal (strep) infections and require an antibiotic. Still, it's important to know which kind of sore throat you're nursing. You might have strep throat if you have most of the following symptoms:

- A sudden, severe sore throat
- A fever over 101°F
- White or yellow spots in the back of a bright red throat
- Headache and/or stomach pain
- Absence of stuffy nose or signs of a cold—in fact, the most distinguishing factor of strep is that there are almost NEVER any signs of a cold, such as a stuffy nose or cough.

If your health care provider does a "rapid strep test" and you have strep throat, you'll be given a prescription for antibiotics. The antibiotics help prevent the infection from spreading to other people and will also reduce the risk of spreading it to other parts of your body, such as your heart. Newer research shows that, for many people, a three- to six-day course of antibiotics is as effective as the traditional ten-day treatment. However, you should take the antibiotics exactly as they are prescribed to ensure that you've adequately defeated the bacteria.

Penicillin is highly effective and inexpensive, and untreated strep throat can lead to rheumatic heart disease, so I'm not advocating for using herbs instead of antibiotics. But for those of you who are interested, echinacea not only revs up the immune system, making it better able to fend off an infection, but a 2009 study from the University of British Columbia found that it readily inactivates

S. pyogenes, the bacteria that causes strep throat. And barberry, along with other berberine-rich herbs like goldenseal, blocks the attachment of *S. pyogenes* to our cells, reducing infection.

WARNING: Do not use berberine-containing plants if you are pregnant or breast-feeding.

Always take a probiotic while taking antibiotics to reduce the risk of antibiotic-associated diarrhea and yeast infection. The following strains of probiotics have been clinically shown to be effective at the doses provided and can be found in many pharmacies and almost all health food stores/natural grocers. Take these at least two hours apart from the antibiotic, and continue to take them for seven days after completing your treatment.

For children up to 12 years of age:

- *Saccharomyces boulardii:* 250 milligrams twice a day
- *Lactobacillus* GG: 1 billion colony-forming units once a day

For people 12 years and older:

- *Saccharomyces boulardii:* 500 milligrams twice a day
- *Lactobacillus* GG: 1 billion colony-forming units twice a day

✚ Seek Medical Attention Now for Sore Throat Symptoms

- If you have the sudden onset of a sore throat, with fever and no signs of a cold (this could indicate strep throat)
- If you develop a fever one to two days after feeling better
- If you develop a skin rash
- If you develop painful joints
- If you have shortness of breath or chest pain
- If your urine is very dark
- If you are unable to swallow and take in fluids

▶ Seasonal Allergies

Spring is one of my favorite seasons. I love to see the first signs of green poking through the soil. But spring is also the time of year when people's allergies start acting up. The trees are blooming, the pollen takes flight, and the annual ritual of itchy eyes and sneezing begins again. Roughly 35 million Americans live with seasonal allergic rhinitis, or what we commonly call hay fever.

As we discussed in the introduction to this chapter, the nose acts as a filter, trapping pollen and other small particles to prevent them from getting into the lungs. During the windy spring months, that means the nose is hard at work, trapping all kinds of pollen and particles. If you don't suffer from allergies, you

R℞ PRESCRIPTION FROM DR. LOW DOG
The Hygiene Hypothesis

In affluent, Western countries, there is far more allergic disease than in developing countries with large, rural populations. And in affluent nations, there is far more allergic disease in urban settings than in rural farming areas. These findings led researchers in the 1980s to propose the "hygiene hypothesis," which suggests that exposure to germs in childhood primes and trains the immune system, protecting against asthma, allergies, eczema, and possibly even autoimmune disorders later in life. Now, almost 40 years later, we've learned that vaccinations, early antibiotic use, antibacterial soaps, urban environment, and C-section birth can all increase the risk of allergic diseases, while growing up with siblings, early day care, a rural environment, and childhood infections appear to be protective. Take-home message: Our innate defense system evolved in a world filled with microbes and germs. The more we eliminate them from our lives, the more our immune system sees food, pollen, and even our own cells as dangerous and foreign.

will hardly notice. It's only when potentially dangerous substances are inhaled that the nose swells to block their entry. The eyes have a similar defense mechanism. If they sense something harmful, they begin to water to flush it out.

But for people with seasonal allergic rhinitis, their bodies perceive harmless pollens as dangerous and react accordingly. Immune cells mount an attack against the allergens, just like they would if the allergens were bacteria or viruses. Chemicals like histamine are released, causing you to sneeze, your nose to run, and your eyes to water.

This same allergic response can happen on a bigger scale if someone is allergic to an insect bite or particular food. In some cases, like a bee sting or peanut allergy, anaphylaxis—the most severe form of allergic reaction—can occur. Treatment involves administration of epinephrine to prevent the throat from swelling shut. (More on this subject is found in the section on bug bites.)

This type of severe reaction doesn't happen with seasonal allergies, but make no mistake: It can make you feel pretty miserable. The good news is that you can use a number of natural remedies to ease your symptoms!

Nasal Irrigation

Allergists are increasingly recommending buffered saline nasal wash using a neti pot. That's because studies have shown a 27 percent improvement in nasal symptoms and a 62 percent reduction in medicine consumption in people who practice this simple procedure! That's dramatic when you think about it! If I can convince someone to do it every single day for at least two weeks, they never fail to come back to the office saying how much better they feel. If I could give you only one recommendation, it'd be to use saline washes regularly. See the recipe and instructions earlier in this chapter, on pages 84–86.

Quercetin

When we have an allergic reaction to something, "mast cells" degranulate, which means they release histamine and other chemicals that cause your nose to get stuffy, your eyes to itch, and in more severe cases, the smooth muscle in your lungs to constrict. A natural compound called quercetin, found in many plants, including citrus fruits, dark berries, and red wine, has been shown to stabilize the membranes of mast cells and to reduce the release of histamine. Although eating more of these foods in your diet might help, I've found quercetin to be very useful if taken regularly at the start of the allergy season if you really suffer from allergies. The dose is generally 500 milligrams twice a day.

Note: Although considered safe, the use of quercetin in pregnancy, particularly at these doses, is not recommended.

Butterbur

Butterbur *(Petasites hybridus)* is a large-leaved plant that was used for centuries in Europe, northern Africa, and Asia to relieve coughs, congestion, and asthma. Scientists have found compounds in the plant that reduce smooth muscle constriction in the lungs and shrink swollen nasal membranes, providing evidence for its historical uses. European clinical trials have shown that butterbur is as effective as leading allergy medications.

Allergies can aggravate asthma, and butterbur can help here, as well. A study of 64 adults and 16 children at the Heidelberg University in Germany reported a decrease in the number, duration, and severity of asthma attacks during two months of butterbur therapy, compared to a baseline. Butterbur extracts are not sedating and are very well tolerated in both kids and adults.

Purchase a product standardized to provide 7.5 milligrams petasin per 50 milligrams of extract and FREE of pyrrolizidine alkaloids. Take 1 capsule morning and night (100 milligrams total each day). Children 6 to 9 years should take 25 milligrams twice a day, while children 9 to 13 take 50 milligrams twice a day.

Note: Because we don't know the safety of butterbur in pregnancy, I'd avoid it.

Nettle Leaf

The dreaded "stinging" nettle *(Urtica dioica)* can pack quite a punch if you rub up against it while out hiking. However, cooking, drying, or making an extract from nettles turns the leaves sting-free! Researchers have found that compounds within nettle leaves inhibit the release of histamine, which causes nasal swelling and itching. A randomized trial of nearly 100 people found that taking 600 milligrams a day of freeze-dried nettle was more effective than placebo for relieving the majority of allergy symptoms. Forty-eight percent of the participants stated that nettles equaled or surpassed previous medications that they had taken for seasonal allergies in terms of effectiveness.

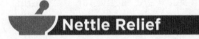

Nettle Relief

20 grams nettle leaf, fresh is best
100 milliliters vodka (80 to 100 proof)

Carefully put nettles into a widemouthed jar and add vodka. Let it sit, covered, and shake daily for 2 weeks. Strain through muslin cloth, pour decanted liquid into a dark bottle, label, and store. Compost herbs.

How to Use: Take ½ teaspoon 2 to 3 times a day.

You can purchase freeze-dried nettles in capsules. The dose is 300 milligrams 2 to 3 times a day. If you live where nettles grow, you can wear gloves and carefully gather them. Let them wilt overnight. Then tincture them in the morning.

✚ Seek Immediate Medical Attention if Your Allergic Reaction Causes:

- Wheezing or difficulty breathing
- Swelling of the lips, eyes, tongue, or mouth
- Chest pain and tightness
- Shock or sudden loss of consciousness
- Hives or joint swelling
- Widespread, intense skin redness
- Nausea, vomiting, or abdominal cramps

If you live in a remote area, keep an epinephrine auto-injector around (for example, EpiPen, Twinject). These can be lifesaving in cases of acute anaphylactic (severe allergic) reactions.

❯ Cold Sores

If you suffer from cold sores, you know the sign of an impending breakout: that slight tingling or numbness near your lip. "Oh, no . . . not now," you say to yourself. Cold sores, also called fever blisters, always seem to show up at the most inopportune times, usually when you have somewhere important to go or something important to do. I know, because I get cold sores, and they're embarrassing, so I've spent years looking into treatments that will quicken the healing time.

Cold sores are caused by herpes simplex virus type 1 (HSV-1). They're more common than you might think: Roughly 85 percent of Americans have been infected with the virus by the time they turn 50 years old.

The name "herpes" comes from the Greek *herpein*, which means "to creep" or a "creeping thing." (That's why people who study snakes are called herpetologists.) Transmitted by personal contact, the virus enters the body through the skin or mucus membrane. From there, it "creeps" up the nerves until it reaches the "terminal nerve cluster" in the spinal cord. Once there, it resides for life, lying dormant until reactivated by a weakness in your immune system.

The virus then starts to multiply and "creeps" back down the nerve pathways. At this point, it can be spread to others, even though the characteristic blisters and sores don't develop for hours or days. The ensuing eruption consists of several tiny

R X — PRESCRIPTION FROM DR. LOW DOG
Is It a Cold Sore or a Canker Sore?

Patients often come to me wondering if the painful ulcer-like disruptions on the inside of the lips or cheeks or under the tongue are cold sores. No—they're canker sores, characterized by a red color with a whitish or whitish yellow coating. Canker sores are unrelated to cold sores.

No one knows exactly what causes canker sores, but being tired or stressed, undergoing trauma, or eating acidic foods such as tomatoes and pineapple have all been linked to outbreaks. Canker sores can be a symptom of sensitivity to gluten (the protein found in many grains), celiac disease, or B_{12} deficiency.

Treatments other than drugs can help. The Sage Gargle listed in "Sore Throat Soothers" (on page 111) works really well, as does propolis, myrrh, or licorice tincture applied with a cotton swab directly on the canker sore four to six times a day. However, if you have frequent canker sores or whitish patches in your mouth that don't go away within 10 to 14 days, make sure you consult your health care provider. If you have recurrent canker sores, you should ask about being tested for celiac.

blisters that eventually congregate to form one large sore around the lips or nose. Some of the common triggers are colds and fevers (hence the name), excessive exposure to the sun, physical trauma, and emotional stress.

HSV-1 is spread through casual contact, so it's almost impossible to prevent. After all, who wants to go through life avoiding kisses? And so often, we share personal items such as cups or silverware, without evening thinking about it. Are there some practical measures you can take to reduce future outbreaks and to shorten them if they occur? Definitely. Here's what I personally use and recommend to my patients:

- *Wear sunblock or sunscreen.* If you spend time on the beach or on the ski slopes, reapply frequently to your lips.
- *Get a new toothbrush.* Toothbrushes can harbor the virus, so make sure you trade yours in at the end of an outbreak.
- *Take your zinc.* Studies show that salivary zinc levels are low during an acute outbreak and lower in those who have recurrent infections. Make sure you are getting 15 to 30 milligrams of zinc glycinate or zinc gluconate every day, and take zinc lozenges during acute outbreaks.
- *Consider lysine.* For more protection, supplement with lysine, an essential amino acid found in meat, poultry, and dairy. There is evidence that taking 500 to 1,000 milligrams of lysine a day can reduce the frequency and severity of recurrent outbreaks. Some experts advise taking 3,000 milligrams a day during acute outbreaks; however, these larger doses should be used only for 7 to 10 days.
- *Manage stress.* Easier said than done! But I know I'm much more vulnerable to having cold sores return when I'm tired and run-down. Do the things you know are good for you: regular exercise, plenty of sleep, and meditation.

R℞ PRESCRIPTION FROM DR. LOW DOG
Genital Herpes

Genital herpes is similar to cold sores, but the eruptions appear in the genital area. It is almost always caused by HSV-2, but also can be caused by HSV-1, usually spread through oral sex. In fact, HSV-1 is thought to be the culprit in half of all the new cases of genital herpes. HSV-2 can also cause oral herpes, though this is less common.

To reduce your risk of genital herpes, do not engage in sex during an active outbreak. Blisters do not have to be visible for you or your partner to be contagious, however. Use a latex condom while having intercourse. Natural condoms made from animal skin (such as lamb) allow the viral particles to pass through them. Use a dental dam if engaging in oral sex. My suggestions for the prevention and treatment of cold sores apply to genital herpes as well.

Licorice

Here is my favorite go-to remedy for cold sores. I cannot tell you the number of times I've used licorice tincture when I felt that old familiar tingle, usually before a big presentation or important event. And it's always the same result: The vast majority of the time, the blisters never even appear.

Why does licorice work so well? According to some scientific investigations, licorice root has compounds that block the virus from creeping down the nerves and causing eruptions on the surface tissue. Licorice also has powerful anti-inflammatory effects that reduce redness and swelling. Licorice tincture therefore offers multiple defenses for attacking the outbreak. Incidentally, I prefer a tincture to tea, because the alcohol disrupts the envelope of the herpes virus, which speeds healing. See my recipe for Licorice Relief Tincture in "The Eighteen Essentials," page 285.

Lemon Balm

Lemon balm extract is made from the herb *Melissa officinalis*. In research, creams containing this herb have been shown to reduce the duration and severity of cold sores when applied topically several times a day soon after they appear. You can purchase these creams at natural grocery stores or online. Or, just put a drop of lemon balm essential oil directly on the blister three times a day for one to two days. This treatment can be quite effective, but be careful with undiluted essential oil, as it can cause irritation if used too long or on sensitive skin.

Chapter 4

Calming the Nerves, Strengthening the Nervous System

The human nervous system is an exquisitely complex information highway that controls all of our biological processes, movements, and thoughts. Because of its vast reach in the body, I feel it is important to focus in on one primary area—how the body responds to stress. Let's start by quickly familiarizing ourselves with how the nervous system is organized.

The central nervous system (CNS) is made up of the brain and spinal cord. The brain is responsible for processing complex information, and the spinal cord serves as a relay for bringing messages to and from the brain. The peripheral nervous system is comprised of the somatic nervous system and the autonomic nervous system (ANS). The somatic nervous system is responsible for transmitting all the messages coming from our skeletal muscles and sensory organs. The ANS is in charge of all the "automatic" functions in our body, things we don't consciously control like the secretion of stomach acid or the beating of our heart. I am primarily interested in discussing the ANS, because it is the part of our nervous system so intimately involved with stress.

The ANS is divided into two parts, the parasympathetic nervous system (PSNS) and the sympathetic nervous system (SNS). The ANS takes its orders from the hypothalamus and pituitary, master controllers located in the brain. The sympathetic response is quick—think of it like a gas pedal in your car. It is responsible for the "fight-or-flight" response, for handling emergencies.

The SNS has direct control over the cells located in the adrenal medulla that secrete epinephrine (adrenaline) and norepinephrine (noradrenaline) to increase heart rate, blood pressure, and blood sugar and shut down digestion and any other systems not essential for immediate survival. These hormones stimulate the pituitary to release hormones that instruct the adrenal cortex to release cortisol. This link is referred to as the hypothalamic-pituitary-adrenal (HPA) axis, as it is a tightly regulated and coordinated system that is unified by the ANS.

Cortisol ramps up the production of blood sugar by the liver, countering the effects of insulin, suppresses parts of the immune system, and shuts down many functions in the body that are not immediately necessary for survival.

But the stress response also has an off switch. The two branches of the ANS work together in a complementary fashion. The parasympathetic interacts with many of the same systems as the SNS in the body, but generally in the opposite direction. Think of it like stepping on the brakes in your car. It slows your heart rate, lowers blood pressure, stimulates digestion, and relaxes you. This is why it's often referred to as the "rest-and-digest" response.

Our body was designed to respond quickly to threats; this was essential for our survival. When the brain detects danger, whether from a charging lion or burglar, it releases hormones that stimulate the SNS to go into action. Stress hormones are released, allowing you to increase your strength and agility, enhance your reflexes, and focus your concentration. The stress response shuts down systems regulating growth, reproduction, metabolism, and immunity. You must divert all your resources to dealing with the threat. When you safely escape the lion's clutches or the police arrive, the parasympathetic system is activated, the stress response is turned off, and your body relaxes.

The problem today, however, is that most of us aren't being chased by lions but by emails, text messages, long hours of work, family demands, financial problems, and so on. There's no off switch for the stress response; we have our foot on the gas all the time. Why does this happen to some and not others? Researchers believe it is genetically driven in part. But as we know, our environment shapes the expression of our genes. Scientists have found that when people are exposed to high levels of stress, particularly in childhood, they maintain an elevated level of cortisol for years. They have an exaggerated response to stressful situations, making them vulnerable to depression, anxiety, and obsessive-compulsive behaviors. Many turn to drugs, alcohol, or food in an attempt to self-medicate these heightened feelings. They have, in effect, lost the ability to "counterregulate" the SNS.

More than 70 million Americans have insomnia. People that persistently have difficulty falling asleep have been found to have higher cortisol levels throughout the first part of the night, when cortisol levels are typically low. Researchers have found that those with the highest blood levels of cortisol had the hardest time falling asleep. At night when they lie down to go to sleep, their stress response is active, telling them to be awake and on the lookout for danger.

It's not that stress is bad. It's our response to it that determines how it will impact our health. What we know is that the consequences of sustained levels of cortisol increase our risk for obesity, heart disease, diabetes, irritable bowel syndrome, heartburn, low libido, infertility, hypothyroidism, infection, delayed healing, and even certain cancers. Scientists believe that prolonged elevation of stress hormones may shorten our life span by 15 years. In effect, what was designed to save our lives has now put us at risk.

In my book *Life Is Your Best Medicine,* I devoted a lot of space to discussing the myriad ways you can increase your resiliency, or your ability to cope with the ups and downs of life. Eating a minimally processed diet, practicing daily meditation, spending time in nature, exercising regularly, listening to music, cultivating healthy relationships, extending forgiveness, and finding contentment all dampen the sympathetic drive. You'll feel calmer and more relaxed, and—no matter what problems you're dealing with in your life—you'll cope more effectively once you have learned to center and ground yourself.

Nothing can replace a healthy diet. The more stressed you are, the more likely you are to go for the junk food and sugar. Although this might temporarily make you feel better, you're fueling the fire. Make a conscious effort to ensure you are getting plenty of healthy protein and avoid high-glycemic-load foods that will just exacerbate blood sugar swings. And if you are under a considerable amount of stress and don't always eat right, you might want to consider taking a multivitamin to ensure that you are getting adequate levels of nutrients to ensure a healthy nervous system. Deficiencies in folate, vitamins B_6 and B_{12}, iron, and zinc can all contribute to fatigue and a depressed mood. Omega-3 fatty acids are also vital for maintaining a healthy mood and countering the adverse effects of stress.

You CAN learn to manage your stress without the use of prescription drugs. In addition to all the lifestyle choices I've listed, I want to share with you the abundance that nature has offered to help us better cope with stress, relieve anxiety, lift our mood, improve our sleep, and ease our pain so that we can fend off many of the more chronic conditions that will need medical intervention.

◐ Resiliency: The Role for Herbal Medicine

Nature has blessed us with many herbs that have a soothing effect upon our nervous system and that help our bodies cope and adapt to stressful situations. I firmly believe that these are needed now more than they've ever been in our history. It is extremely rare for me to see a patient whose health has not been compromised in some way by an inability to deal with stressful people and events in life. This is why I almost always recommend two classes of herbal therapies: nervines and adaptogens.

Nervines

At its most basic definition, a nervine is simply an herb that has some effect upon the nervous system. This category of plants is broken down into three categories, based upon the physiologic effect of the herb.

Nervine stimulants. You probably had a dose this morning. Caffeinated coffee and tea are classic examples of this class. The effects of caffeine vary among individuals and also vary based upon how much you consume. Caffeine causes blood levels of epinephrine and norepinephrine to rise, increases heart rate, elevates cholesterol in heavy consumers, and acts as a diuretic. I seldom recommend the daily use of herbs such as yerba maté, guarana, coffee, or tea, as many people already consume them and most people are already overstimulated.

However, herbs like peppermint, rosemary, and ginger are also nervine stimulants. They enliven and awaken the nervous system without overstimulating. Peppermint is uplifting and energizing. Peppermint tea in the afternoon or evening can help you focus on work or studies without impairing your ability to sleep. The menthol in peppermint can relieve cough and ease congestion. I inhale rosemary essential oil when I am driving long distances, as it keeps my mind sharp and focused. Rosemary, the herb of remembrance, is said to improve memory and concentration.

Nervine relaxants. These are the herbs that have a calming effect upon our nerves. Their effects range from mild and gentle, such as chamomile and lemon balm, to the more powerful sedative plants like hops and California poppy. They free up our resistance, which often presents as irritability, tension, and depression. I rely heavily upon these plants in my practice, choosing the one that most closely fits the person's constitution in my formulations. Here are just a few insights into the personality of a few of the nervine relaxants:

- German chamomile is one of the best herbs for those who hold stress in their digestive tracts and skin. Chamomile's anti-inflammatory activity eases eczema and digestive upset, while its antispasmodic effect quiets irritable bowel. It is the primary herb used for infant colic.
- Lemon balm is for the social butterflies among us who become irritable and cranky when they don't have enough downtime. Lemon balm is for overstimulated extroverts with difficulty focusing, a good choice for kids and adults with ADHD or those that just go and go and go.
- Valerian is found in many sleep formulations because it can help release us into sleep. It is best for those who are tense and tired. It relaxes tension in the muscles, making it a good choice for those with spasms, cramps, and tension headaches.
- California poppy is my go-to herb for those who are stressed-out, depressed, and cannot sleep because of pain. It has mild pain-relieving properties, eases anxiety, and helps induce restful sleep. Effective and safe, it is not addictive like its cousin, the opium poppy.
- Hops are my choice for those who really need to sleep but find themselves lying awake at night worried about

all kinds of things. Hops bind melatonin receptors, which may explain in part why this relaxant works. I once drank 2 cups of very strong hops tea before bed and slept for 10 hours straight. It works.

Nervine tonics. These are herbs that nourish and support the nervous system. We have no equivalent in Western medicine. Traditionally, these remedies were used when there was actual physical damage to the nerves and for those who were emotionally exhausted and overwhelmed. Here are three of my favorites:

- Milky oats is a classic nervine tonic. It is my go-to tonic for those who are mentally and spiritually tired—not depressed, but just spent. I've seen this in many caregivers, healers, and pastors. Milky oats are harvested and tinctured while in their green, milky stage.
- Skullcap is best for those who are easily upset and easily overwhelmed. The old expression, "I am on my last nerve!" accurately describes someone who would benefit from skullcap both acutely and as a tonic. It is one of my top herbs for those who do not handle stress well.
- St. John's wort strengthens and nourishes those who are mildly depressed. A 2009 review of 29 studies concluded that St. John's wort is as effective as standard prescription antidepressants for treating mild to moderate depression. I've found it to be highly beneficial for those who grew up with little sense of personal boundaries, always becoming enmeshed in the emotional needs of others and then feeling overwhelmed and depressed. It's best for those not taking prescription drugs as it can interact with many.

You can make teas or tinctures from these herbs based upon which one resonates with you. On the next page is a recipe for St. John's wort tincture. For young children, stick with chamomile, lemon balm, milky oats, and skullcap. Following is a great

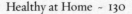
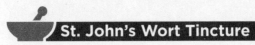

St. John's Wort Tincture

25 grams St. John's wort, fresh flowering tops
65 milliliters grain alcohol
40 milliliters water

To make a 1:5 fresh herb tincture, chop the St. John's wort into small pieces and put them in a jar. Add 65 milliliters grain alcohol and 40 milliliters water to achieve a 1:5 strength fresh herb tincture with a solvency of 50 percent (you have to account for the water in the fresh herb). Mix well. Cover with a lid and label. Steep for 2 to 4 weeks. Strain through a cheesecloth and store in a dark bottle.

How to Use: St. John's wort tincture is a highly effective mood lifter. The dose of tincture for an adult is 3 milliliters 2 to 3 times a day. The tincture may also be applied topically as a compress for bruises and nerve pain.

Although most people think of St. John's wort as the "anti-depressant" herb, the truth is that it has been used for more than 2,000 years to calm the nerves, lift one's mood, and help reduce pain. Modern science has confirmed that it is as effective as prescription antidepressants for mild to moderate depression, and preliminary research also shows it can ease PMS symptoms and improve menopausal symptoms. The one thing you have to watch for when using St. John's wort is possible herb-drug interactions. Check with your pharmacist or health care provider before using it internally if you are taking any prescription medications.

basic stress formula that is great to keep around the house for those times when you need to "take the edge off." In the section titled "Insomnia: Welcoming the Sandman" (pages 134–141), I will show you how to incorporate herbs such as hops and California poppy into it for use as a sleep aid.

Herbal Stress Relief

10 grams lemon balm herb
10 grams chamomile flowers
10 grams skullcap herb
150 milliliters brandy or vodka OR
170 milliliters vegetable glycerin and 70 milliliters water

Grind herbs into a coarse powder and put in a glass jar. Add vodka OR vegetable glycerin and water. Stir well. If you need to add more liquid, put in an additional 15 milliliters glycerin and 5 milliliters water. Cover and let sit for 2 weeks, shaking daily. Strain and pour liquid into a dark bottle, label, and store in a cabinet. Compost herbs.

How to Use:
Herbal Stress Relief Tincture (made with brandy or vodka):
Teens and adults: Take 1 teaspoon of the tincture 2 to 3 times a day, as needed to ease tension or anxiety.

Herbal Stress Relief Glycerite:
40 to 60 pounds: $1/2$ teaspoon 2 to 3 times a day, as needed
60 to 90 pounds: 1 teaspoon 2 to 3 times a day, as needed
90 to 120 pounds: $1 1/2$ teaspoons 2 to 3 times a day, as needed
Over 120 pounds: 2 teaspoons 2 to 3 times a day, as needed

Adaptogens

Adaptogens are the other category of herb that should have a prominent place in our modern herbal pharmacy. Soviet researchers coined the term back in the 1960s, while looking for substances that could increase the work productivity of laborers, soldiers, and scientists without causing them harm. Much of their early research had been conducted on Asian ginseng and eleuthero, previously known as Siberian ginseng. They found that these herbs could increase nonspecific resistance, meaning they seemed to enhance resiliency in those who took them.

Today, we know that these herbs work on the hypothalamic-pituitary-adrenal (HPA) axis, modulating the effects of the autonomic nervous system. Given the rapidly growing body of evidence that shows the long-term consequences of persistently elevated cortisol, I believe there is a definite place for these herbs in our lives.

Over the last 20 years, I have increasingly used adaptogens in my practice and have seen amazing results when taken over time. Although there are many adaptogens, I would like to share just a few of my favorites with you.

- Ginseng is considered by many to be the classic adaptogen. In traditional Chinese medicine, Asian ginseng is prescribed for those with low energy, a tendency to feel cold, and a lack of sex drive. Studies have shown ginseng improves erectile dysfunction in men and mood and quality of life in women transitioning through menopause. Studies suggest it may reduce the frequency of colds and have a beneficial effect on blood sugar in people with diabetes. Not surprising, ginseng has been shown to lower cortisol when elevated, which may explain the myriad benefits associated with its use.

- Ashwagandha is considered a *rasayana,* or rejuvenating tonic, in Ayurveda, the traditional medical system of India. The species name *somnifera* means "sleep-inducing," hinting at its calming effect. I think of ashwagandha for those who are wired and tired, exhausted by 7 p.m. but unable to sleep and suddenly wide-awake with a racing mind once they lie down. Ashwagandha has been shown to enhance the immune response, making it easier to fend off colds and respiratory infections. It also has a mild stimulating effect on the thyroid gland. A study of 64 people with anxiety found that ashwagandha significantly lowered cortisol levels compared to those taking a placebo. Remember, elevated cortisol can make it hard to fall asleep, can suppress the immune system and thyroid function, and can increase feelings of anxiousness.

- Rhodiola has been used in the traditional medicine systems of eastern Europe and Asia for more than 3,000 years, believed to increase energy, decrease depression, eliminate fatigue, and prevent high-altitude sickness. Multiple studies show it improves depression, while a UCLA study found it improved symptoms of generalized anxiety disorder. A Scandinavian study found that it improved chronic fatigue. This is my go-to herb for those with fatigue, mental fog, maybe a bit of depression, and

Tieraona's Winter Elixir

10 grams ashwagandha root
10 grams rhodiola root
10 grams astragalus root
150 milliliters brandy or vodka plus 2 tablespoons honey OR
170 milliliters vegetable glycerin plus 70 milliliters water

Grind herbs into a coarse powder and put in glass jar. Add brandy, vodka, OR vegetable glycerin and water. Stir well. If you need to add more liquid, put in an additional 30 milliliters brandy or vodka or 25 milliliters glycerin and 5 milliliters water. Cover with a lid and let sit for 2 weeks, shaking daily. Strain and pour liquid into a dark bottle, label, and store in a cabinet. Compost herbs.

How to Use: Take 1 teaspoon brandy or vodka elixir or 2 teaspoons glycerin elixir every day.

I include astragalus to give me a little extra immune protection during the winter. You can leave this out and just use 15 grams of rhodiola and ashwagandha.

difficulty concentrating. I have had patients with chronic fatigue syndrome and fibromyalgia tell me it worked wonders for them.

You might find taking one of these adaptogens helpful if you're feeling under a great deal of stress. I generally recommend them for a period of two to three months, long enough to get the benefits. Can you take them longer? Well, yes, but they should be part of a holistic approach to managing stress. I don't think it's wise to use an herb or a drug in place of doing all the things that will allow us to experience good health.

Having said that, I almost always take an adaptogen-rich elixir during the winter to help me counteract the stressful effects of extensive traveling, as winter is my busiest time of year for attending and teaching at conferences. I find that the elixir helps me sleep better, fend off illness, and handle lost luggage, cranky passengers, and a houseful of relatives with relative ease!

▶ Insomnia: Welcoming the Sandman

From waking to nurse my babies, being on call at the hospital, staying up to catch a baby, to now, frequently traveling across time zones, I have spent most of my adult life getting by on little sleep. Even on the nights when I am at home in my own bed, sleep can prove elusive. I often awaken around three or four in the morning and find it hard to go back to sleep. I admit, however, that I often enjoy those early mornings. The house is quiet and it feels like a magical time to read or write while sipping on hot tea. Every few nights, my body will feel tired and I enjoy a restful night's sleep.

I'm not alone when it comes to sleepless nights. Roughly half of all Americans struggle with occasional insomnia. You might not be sleeping well for many reasons, too many to cover in this section. If you give these sleep remedies a try and nothing seems to help, that's the time to check in with your health care provider to see if a sleep study or other evaluation might be a useful next step. However, the vast majority of insomnia is due to lifestyle choices and stress. And what's more, chronic stress and insomnia can lead to many unhealthy daytime behaviors that further aggravate both problems. When tired, people often consume more caffeine and high-sugar/high-fat foods in an attempt to feel more energetic. Individuals are also less likely to exercise because they feel "too tired." Insomnia decreases one's ability to concentrate and focus, making job and school performance suffer. More alarming, it may increase the risk for heart disease and obesity. Studies published in leading medical journals suggest that sleep loss may increase hunger and affect the body's metabolism, making it more difficult to maintain or lose weight.

The good news, though, is that you can do many, many things to manage your stress and improve sleep.

Practical Tips

Light. The timing and type of light we're exposed to can have a dramatic influence on our sleep. Exposure to natural daylight is vitally important for keeping your internal clock in sync. The blue light of the sun suppresses the production of melatonin, telling your body it is time to be up and awake. As night begins to fall, it's just as important to start dimming the lights so your melatonin levels begin to rise. Dimmer switches on lamps and lights are a great way to accomplish this. Either commit to turning off your computers and mobile devices two to three hours before bed or install software that will shift from blue light to red light as evening approaches. (F.lux is one example of free software that you can use.) Invest in blackout curtains or thick drapes to shut out light at night and, if you're a light sleeper, use a fan or white noise machine to drown out traffic, barking dogs, and so on.

R℞ PRESCRIPTION FROM DR. LOW DOG
Dawn and Dusk Simulation

I have found that, although primarily used for people living with seasonal affective disorder, dawn and dusk simulation devices can be extremely helpful for those with sleep problems. At night, the light gradually fades as you fall asleep, mimicking sunset, and in the morning, about 20 to 40 minutes before it is time to wake up, the light gets brighter, simulating sunrise. Most have white noise available, which can help block out noise at night. I absolutely love mine and have recommended it to patients, and have given them as gifts to family members and friends.

Alcohol. If you're waking up in the middle of the night and are having a hard time going back to sleep, it might be that second glass of wine you had with dinner! Although alcohol may help you fall asleep, it prevents you from going into the deepest stages of sleep, leaving you awake at night and tired in the morning. For two weeks, don't drink any alcohol within three hours of going to bed and limit yourself to no more than one serving if you're a woman and two servings if you're a man.

Exercise. Many people exercise at night after work, because it's the only time in the day that really works. But exercise gets your adrenaline pumping and raises your body temperature, exactly the opposite of what you want to fall asleep. If you're having a problem sleeping and you exercise in the evening, do a two-week trial of not exercising within three hours of bedtime. In other words, if you want to be in bed sleeping by 10 p.m., finish your workout by 7 p.m.

Medication check. Many medications can interfere with sleep. Drugs used to treat high blood pressure, heart disease, asthma, allergies, and depression are a few of the categories known to be problematic. You can usually take other options, so make sure to talk to your health care provider and/or pharmacist.

Snoring. If someone has told you that you snore or snort at night and you wake up feeling tired most mornings—you might have a condition called sleep apnea. Treatments are available so tell your physician about your symptoms and ask if a sleep study would be right for you.

Restless legs. Restless leg syndrome (RLS) is a neurological condition characterized by unpleasant sensations (for example, crawling, creeping, pulling) in the legs and an overwhelming need to move them, particularly when trying to relax. The cause is not entirely known, but iron, folic acid, or magnesium deficiency can bring it on. Stretching and yoga postures can be very helpful, as can 400 to 600 milligrams of magnesium taken at night before bed. If symptoms persist, talk to your primary care provider.

Natural Remedies for Sleep

You can use a number of remedies to help you sleep better at night. But don't expect miracles if you're racing 100 miles an hour until your head hits the pillow and then you think a tincture or pill is going to magically knock you out. Medicines that can do that are almost always addictive and have side effects. The key is to prepare for sleep by getting plenty of sunshine and exercise during the day, eating lightly in the evening, and slowing down around two hours before bed.

I've been making my own Slumber Elixir for almost 20 years now and have found that taking it consistently for at least 10 to 12 days helps about 80 percent of those who use it to fall asleep faster and stay asleep longer. I've used it in children as

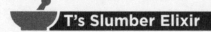

T's Slumber Elixir

5 grams hops flowers
5 grams valerian root
5 grams California poppy herb
5 grams lemon balm herb
100 milliliters brandy and 2 tablespoons honey OR
115 milliliters vegetable glycerin and 45 milliliters water

Grind the herbs and put in a tall glass jar. Add brandy and honey OR vegetable glycerin and water. Stir well. If you need more alcohol, add another 20 milliliters brandy. If making a glycerite, add an additional 15 milliliters vegetable glycerin and 5 milliliters water.

Cover with a lid and let sit for 2 weeks. Strain and put in a dark bottle, label, and store in a cabinet. Compost herbs.

How to Use:
Slumber Elixir with brandy:
Teens and adults: Take 1 to 1½ teaspoons 30 minutes before bed. Can be taken in hot water, tea, juice, or straight off the spoon.

Slumber Elixir with glycerin:
60 to 90 pounds: 1 teaspoon 30 minutes before bed
90 to 120 pounds: 1½ to 2 teaspoons 30 minutes before bed
over 120 pounds: 2 to 3 teaspoons 30 minutes before bed

This can be taken in hot water, tea, juice, or straight off the spoon.

Note: This elixir is designed to help you sleep. Do not take it if you are going to be driving or doing other things that require your attention. Don't mix herbal sedatives with prescription sleeping pills. Women who are pregnant or breast-feeding should not use this elixir.

young as six who were in pain or deeply distraught, though I generally use this for teens and adults with chronic sleep problems. The combination of valerian and hops has been shown to improve sleep in adults, while the combination of valerian and lemon balm was effective for children under the age of 12. Some people find that valerian has a paradoxically stimulating effect. It's not common but can occur, especially in people who have very active minds and imagination. If you think that might be you, leave it out and increase the hops or California poppy to 10 grams. California poppy relieves tension and helps reduce aches and pains that may be preventing a good night's sleep.

Melatonin

Melatonin is a hormone made by your body's pineal gland that is part of your internal clock. During the day, melatonin is barely detectable. As darkness falls, the pineal gland begins to secrete melatonin. Your body temperature begins to slightly drop, you feel less alert, and you get ready for sleep. Melatonin levels stay elevated for 10 to 12 hours, falling as the sun rises.

People with delayed sleep phase syndrome have difficulty falling asleep until late at night or early in the morning. Think teenagers! Studies show that both melatonin and early morning bright light exposure can be helpful for correcting this type of sleep problem in kids and adults.

Europe recently approved a prescription of 2 milligrams sustained-release melatonin for sleep problems in those over the age of 55 years. Some studies suggest that melatonin may be more effective for the elderly, who typically secrete less melatonin. Data from clinical studies showed that melatonin is quite safe when taken up to a year, does not cause rebound insomnia when discontinuing it, and does not suppress the body's natural production of melatonin.

Melatonin has also been shown to relieve heartburn in randomized controlled trials. This might make it the optimal sleep remedy for those with both insomnia and GERD. For more information, see the section on heartburn in Chapter 5.

Doses as low as 0.3 milligram of rapid- or sustained-release melatonin taken 2 hours before bed (when possible, if you're home and not going back out) can be helpful. I usually recommend 1 to 3 milligrams sustained-release melatonin for at least 30 days before deciding whether or not it is going to be helpful.

Magnesium and Calcium

Taking your magnesium and calcium before bed can be a winning combination for those with muscle tension and difficulty sleeping. Take 300 milligrams calcium and 300 milligrams magnesium about 30 to 45 minutes before bed.

L-theanine

L-theanine is a nonprotein amino acid that occurs naturally in the tea plant (Camellia sinensis) and contributes to its pleasant taste. In Japan and other Asian countries, it is widely used to treat anxiety symptoms and depressed mood, and its popularity is growing in the United States. Small studies have shown that L-theanine can enhance relaxation and improve concentration, an effect that lasts for about eight hours. This is consistent with what many consumers of green tea experience, a calm state of heightened alertness, versus the more hyperalert state many experience with coffee. I typically recommend L-theanine throughout the day for those who have difficulty sleeping because of tension and worry.

Take 100 to 200 milligrams 2 to 3 times a day for tension and anxiety and to promote better sleep at night.

||||||||||||||||||||||||||||||||||||||||||||||||||||||||||||||||||||||||||||||||||||||||||||||||||||||||

☎ Call Your Health Care Provider

- If your insomnia lasts for more than four weeks after implementing lifestyle strategies
- If your insomnia makes it difficult for you to stay awake or function during the day

||||||||||||||||||||||||||||||||||||||||||||||||||||||||||||||||||||||||||||||||||||||||||||||||||||||||

▶ Pounding, Splitting, Throbbing: Natural Headache Helpers

I remember the first time I had a migraine. I was driving my daughter to school one morning when I started noticing that everything in the outer edge of my vision looked watery. A few minutes later, I started seeing squiggly flashes of light. I had no head pain, only this dramatic change in my vision. The sensation was startling.

I pulled my car over and called a friend to pick us up. About the time he arrived, my head started to throb. I felt waves of nausea. The sunlight felt excruciating.

My friend took me to the hospital where I was poked, prodded, and scanned. The ER doctor, a friend of mine, said, "Good news, Tieraona, you're not having a stroke. It looks like you're just having a migraine."

JUST a migraine! *Wow.* He'd obviously never had one. Of course, neither had I. It took several days to return to normal.

For the next few years, I was plagued with migraines. I tried lots of measures to get them under control. I kept a strict food and headache diary to see what might be triggering them. I then eliminated those triggers. And I used some very simple measures, which I shall share later in this chapter. I'm happy to report that my migraines are under very good control today.

Headaches are one of the most common pain conditions that prompt people to see a doctor. We doctors classify headaches into two major categories: primary and secondary. Primary headaches are caused by an overactivity of pain-sensitive nerves in the head and include migraine, tension, and cluster headaches.

Secondary headaches are symptoms of an underlying disease, such as infection, concussion, hangover, stroke, meningitis, and so forth. Secondary headaches almost always require a medical evaluation (see the sections about when to seek medical attention, pages 146 and 149), so I'm going to focus on tension and migraine headaches here, because they are the most common and respond favorably to home treatment.

Tension-type headaches are by far the most common type of headache. And although muscle tension may be the culprit in some cases, scientists don't know what causes the majority of them. Environmental, emotional, and physical stressors can trigger them, as can certain medications. Tension headaches can last as little as 30 minutes or linger for days. They are more common in women than men.

Migraine headaches are the second most common painful headache disorder, affecting 10 percent or more of the general population, and are three times more common in women than in men. Migraines are characterized by headache pain on one side of the head, pulsating in quality, and lasting 4 to 70 hours. They are accompanied by sensitivity to light and sound, as well as nausea and vomiting. Some people experience an "aura," a neurological symptom, before or right as the pain begins. The aura is usually visual—for example, you might see flickering lights—but can be motor, such as difficulty speaking, or sensory, like feeling pins and needles. The aura develops gradually, 5 to 20 minutes just before or at the onset of a migraine, is fully reversible, and generally disappears within 60 minutes.

If you are one of those individuals who rarely ever get a headache, then the occasional use of acetaminophen, aspirin, or ibuprofen is reasonable. However, if you're having headaches more often than you'd like, the first step in getting better is to figure out what's triggering them. A headache diary can be really useful. Use a simple notebook, in which you write down what you eat and drink, how long you slept, stressful events, medications, and any headache pain. This information can help you identify your triggers.

Some of the most common triggers are:

Medications. Drugs for depression, high blood pressure, and hormones are all known culprits. And, if you've been taking pain-relieving medications frequently, you can get what's called a "medication overuse" headache. This is a vicious trap because the meds you're using to treat your headaches can actually cause them when used on a regular basis.

Food and food additives. Some studies show that up to 80 percent of migraine sufferers experience some improvement when certain foods or food additives are removed from their diet. Although this list is not exhaustive, and you may be sensitive to none or several of these, the following list is a good place to start looking for food triggers:

- Nitrites and nitrates used to preserve processed meats (hot dogs, deli meats, bacon, pepperoni, and so forth) and many other food products. These are a problem for a lot of folks with headaches.
- Sulfites are often used as a preservative in dried fruits such as prunes, figs, raisins, and apricots; red and white wine; and processed foods. Read labels carefully. Sulfites are a major headache trigger.
- Alcohol is a vasodilator (it widens blood vessels) and a diuretic. Many types of alcohol contain chemicals called congeners. Congeners bestow the specific taste that makes each alcohol unique and are responsible for hangover effects. All these factors make alcohol a formidable trigger.
- Aged cheeses are high in tyramine, a substance that forms from the breakdown of protein in certain foods.

The longer a food ages, the greater the tyramine content. Watch out for aged cheeses such as Brie, cheddar, Muenster, Parmesan, blue cheese, Stilton, Gorgonzola, and processed cheeses. Red wine, pickles, onions, avocados, and olives also fall into this category.

- Chocolate can be a problem for some poor souls! That's because it contains the amino acid phenylethylamine, a known headache trigger.
- Aspartame, a common artificial sweetener, can be a problem. It is used in many diet sodas and snacks.
- Citrus fruits and juices (usually, ½ cup a day is not a problem).
- Caffeine is a mild vasoconstrictor and has been shown to increase the effectiveness of pain and migraine medications. But it can also cause caffeine rebound headaches. If you suffer from headaches, limit your intake to 200 milligrams a day (about two cups of coffee). Some headache sufferers, however, may need to avoid it altogether.
- Monosodium glutamate (MSG) is a salt form of an amino acid used in food preservation and flavoring. MSG can trigger headaches in susceptible people. It is frequently added to Asian dishes, processed meats, and canned goods.

Low blood sugar. Many people report headaches after skipping meals. This may happen because certain hormones are released when blood sugar falls, adversely affecting the contraction of blood vessels. Eating regular meals is key to keeping headaches at bay.

Muscle problems. Tight muscles can be a trigger, particularly in the neck and eyes. Eyestrain can be a big problem, so make sure to have your vision checked regularly. Hot baths, muscle rubs, massage therapy, chiropractic manipulation, and acupuncture are all helpful. If you have chronic muscle and/or joint problems, find what works best for you. This will involve some trial and error, but it's worth it.

Light. Migraine sufferers are often sensitive to light, especially glare. Bright, flickering lights are particularly bad. Use full-spectrum bulbs that mimic natural daylight and antiglare screens on computer displays to reduce flicker. Invest in a good pair of Polaroid sunglasses to reduce glare from snow, sand, and water.

Stress. This is the biggest trigger for headaches. Stress can be environmental and include such triggers as strong odors or chemicals; physical (fatigue is a good example); or emotional, such as worry, anxiety, or depression. When under stress, the body releases chemicals that cause changes in blood vessels that can trigger a migraine or tension headache. The headaches often become more frequent during periods of high stress. After a stressful event or time, the letdown itself can trigger a headache. Developing healthy coping strategies is so important—meditation, yoga, exercise, or whatever works best for you. The Herbal Stress Relief tincture/glycerite in the "Resiliency" section (page 131) can be used by anyone who's feeling stressed.

Menstruation and menopause. Due to falling estrogen levels, women often experience more intense migraines right before and during the first two days of their menstrual period and also during their menopausal years. Some women find the herb chasteberry *(Vitex agnus-castus)* to be helpful during this transition.

▶ Head Off the Hurt: Top Remedies for Headaches

Please Pass the Butterbur

This broad-leaved plant was once used to wrap butter prior to refrigeration, hence its unusual name. Butterbur has been well studied for the prevention of migraine headaches in both children and adults. As a matter of fact, it is now a first-line recommendation for migraine prophylaxis by the American Academy of Neurology, the American Headache Society, and the Canadian Headache Society. That's a strong endorsement for an herbal medicine!

I strongly recommend taking butterbur extract along with magnesium for anyone suffering from migraines. You cannot make the extract at home because butterbur contains small amounts of pyrrolizidine alkaloids, compounds that can damage the liver over time.

Purchase a product standardized to provide 7.5 milligrams petasin per 50 milligrams of extract and FREE of pyrrolizidine alkaloids:

- Take 3 capsules a day for 30 days (150 milligrams a day) and then 1 capsule each morning and night (100 milligrams a day).
- Children 6 to 9 years should take 25 milligrams twice a day.
- Children 9 to 13 take 50 milligrams twice a day.

Because we don't know the safety of butterbur in pregnancy, I'd recommend avoiding it.

||||||||||||||||||||||||||||||||||||||||||||||||||||||||||||||||||||||||||||||||||||||||||||||||||||||||

☎ Call Your Health Care Provider

If your headaches:

- Occur more frequently than usual
- Are more severe than usual
- Worsen or don't improve with appropriate use of over-the-counter headache relievers
- Prevent you from working, sleeping, or participating in your daily activities

||||||||||||||||||||||||||||||||||||||||||||||||||||||||||||||||||||||||||||||||||||||||||||||||||||||||

The Magnesium Solution

Second to butterbur, magnesium is definitely my migraine remedy of choice. I use it personally, and I recommend it to many of my patients. Magnesium is a natural calmative, relaxing muscles and gently dilating blood vessels. This is why it helps with leg cramps and high blood pressure.

Magnesium can help prevent menstrual-related migraines (and menstrual cramps), as well as tension headaches in children and adults. Studies have shown that people with frequent headaches often have low levels of magnesium in their cells, and taking supplemental magnesium can reduce the frequency and severity of migraines. The Canadian Headache Society gives magnesium a "strong recommendation" for migraine prevention. The few times I've forgotten to take magnesium with me while traveling, I've had a migraine within 72 hours. I'm a believer.

Take 600 milligrams of magnesium glycinate or magnesium citrate before bed. The main side effect of magnesium is loose stools, so if this dose gives you diarrhea, just cut back to 400 milligrams for a few weeks and then try increasing again. The nice thing about taking magnesium before bed is that it can help you sleep better, too. Magnesium is safe in pregnancy.

Note: Magnesium is safe at these doses unless you have a problem with your kidneys. If your doctor has told you that you have poor kidney function or kidney failure, you should NOT take supplemental magnesium without talking to your doctor first.

Riboflavin for Relief

Also referred to as vitamin B_2, riboflavin is commonly used for treating muscle cramps, alleviating burning feet syndrome, and preventing migraine headaches. Studies have shown that taking 400 milligrams a day of riboflavin significantly reduces the number of migraine headache attacks. The American Headache

Society listed it as "probably effective" for migraine prevention and treatment.

Take 400 milligrams of riboflavin a day. It can cause your urine to turn orangish yellow. This is harmless. This dose of riboflavin has not been studied in pregnancy or breast-feeding women.

The Peppermint Promise

Peppermint is a wonderful remedy for headache. A study found that massaging peppermint oil into your temples and forehead was as effective for relieving a tension headache as ibuprofen. You can make a peppermint compress (see the section on compresses) or make this simple massage oil at home.

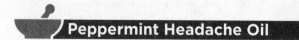

Peppermint Headache Oil

20 drops peppermint essential oil
4 tablespoons (2 ounces) almond, grape seed, or sunflower oil
   as the carrier oil

Put the carrier oil into a bottle and add peppermint essential oil. Shake well. Put on a lid.

How to Use: Gently rub oil into temples, forehead, neck, and shoulders, being careful to avoid the eyes.

Note: Peppermint should not be used on the face of any child under the age of three.

The Fighting Power of Ginger

Ginger is my favorite herb for relieving a tension headache. I'd take it over ibuprofen or aspirin any day. Ginger tea reduces inflammation and relaxes tense muscles. You can also drink it you feel nauseated from a migraine. I strongly suggest keeping a box of medicinal-strength ginger tea bags (look for brands like Traditional Medicinals or Yogi) in your house for times like these. Drink a cup when you first feel a headache coming on. Repeat in an hour or two, if needed.

Feverfew for Migraines?

Although there is some evidence that the herb feverfew can help prevent migraines, I must honestly say that I've had so much more success with butterbur, magnesium, and riboflavin that I just don't recommend it anymore.

 Seek Medical Attention Now for Headaches

- Confusion or trouble understanding speech
- Fainting
- High fever, greater than 103°F, with a stiff neck
- Numbness, weakness, or paralysis on one side of your body
- Trouble seeing, speaking, or walking
- Nausea or vomiting (if not clearly related to the flu or a hangover)
- Headache with a fever, stiff neck, mental confusion, seizures, double vision, weakness, numbness, or speaking difficulties

Chapter 5

Healing the Gut

More than 2,000 years ago, Hippocrates, the famous Greek physician, said that all disease begins in the gut. I'm pretty sure that not all diseases start in the gut but I've found that many conditions improve, to a greater or lesser degree, when gut health is optimized. From heartburn to allergies, it seems many of our woes can be traced to the gastrointestinal (GI) tract. Any gardener knows that healthy soil is absolutely necessary for growing healthy plants. In our bodies, the gut is the soil that allows us to experience vitality and well-being.

▶ The Process

Digestion begins in the mouth. Chewing breaks down food and saliva moistens it to allow for easier swallowing. The salivary glands secrete amylase, an enzyme that starts the breakdown of carbohydrates/starch. Food then travels through the esophagus, the long muscular tube that connects the mouth to the stomach. Here the enzyme gastrin stimulates the release of hydrochloric acid and enzymes like pepsin that break down proteins. The stomach is designed to house a highly acidic environment, with a pH of 2 or less, handily dissolving food and destroying any bacteria or other nasty microbes that enter either through the mouth or travel up from the small intestine. Without sufficient stomach acid, we are more vulnerable to foodborne infections, as well as an overgrowth of bacteria in the small intestine that can cause excess gas and bloating. We also need stomach acid to ensure absorption of iron, copper, zinc, calcium, vitamin B_{12}, folic acid, proteins, and other nutrients.

Gastrin, the hormone released when there's food in the stomach, particularly protein, amino acids, or calcium, is vitally important for digestion and for reducing the risk of heartburn. One of its jobs is to cause the lower esophageal sphincter (LES) to tighten, preventing the backward flow of stomach contents into the sensitive esophagus. It also promotes stomach contractions to move the partially digested food down into the small intestine. The longer foods stay in the stomach, the greater the chance for reflux, gas, and bloating. Our growing love affair with starchy, fatty carbs may be, in part, to blame for all the indigestion people are experiencing. Several studies have shown that a low-carbohydrate diet can eradicate heartburn in many people.

Once the food has been partially digested in the stomach, it enters the first part of the small intestine, the duodenum, where cells secrete the hormones secretin and cholecystokinin (CCK). Secretin triggers the pancreas to release bicarbonate to neutralize stomach acid, and CCK stimulates the liver to release bile and the pancreas to send digestive enzymes. The pancreas actually secretes and releases about eight cups of digestive juices into the small intestine every day. These enzymes neutralize the acid coming from the stomach, and continue to break down fats, proteins, and carbohydrates. Some people cannot manufacture enough enzymes to digest their food. For instance, cystic fibrosis causes the ducts in the pancreas to become clogged with thick mucus, blocking the flow of enzymes into the small intestine. Oral pancreatic enzymes must then be taken to ensure proper nutrition.

The small intestine is where absorption happens, as nutrients, vitamins, and minerals are absorbed through the intestinal wall into the bloodstream. Some conditions, like Crohn's disease, put people at greater risk for nutritional deficiencies because absorption is impaired.

The liver has numerous roles, but one of its primary jobs is to process the nutrients that are absorbed from the small intestine and manufacture many of the chemicals the body needs to survive. The liver is also a major player in the body's innate detoxification processes, breaking down and eliminating harmful chemicals and drugs. Finally, the liver produces bile, which is stored in the gallbladder and released into the small intestine to assist in the digestion of fat. Herbs that stimulate the release of bile from the gallbladder are called cholagogues. They are often used to improve digestion and bowel movements, as bile is a natural laxative.

Waste products are propelled by strong muscular contractions into the large intestine, or colon, and then excreted. It takes roughly 36 hours for stool to pass through the colon. Water is reabsorbed back into the body, making the stool more solid along its journey. The stool is comprised mostly of bacteria and food remains. The colonic bacteria, or microbiota, have many amazing functions, as you will see within the next few pages.

◖ The Second Brain

Our digestive system is complex: It has its own independent nervous system, called the enteric nervous system (ENS). Often referred to as the second brain, the ENS is composed of more than 100 million neurons embedded within the gut wall stretching from the esophagus to the anus. From the mixing and breaking down of food and absorption of nutrients to the rhythmical contractions of the smooth muscles that expel waste, the ENS is the conductor in the symphony that is digestion.

Because the gut is so richly innervated, emotions impact its function. When you feel scared or upset, your brain triggers the release of stress hormones, preparing your body to fight or flee. The ENS responds by slowing or shutting down digestion and elimination. Makes sense, as it would be highly counterproductive to have to stop and go to the bathroom in the middle of a dangerous situation, or waste precious resources on processing dinner. But think about those who live with chronic stress. Shutting down digestive enzymes and inhibiting muscle contractions is a sure setup for gas, bloating, constipation, and irritable bowel syndrome.

The ENS produces neurotransmitters, hormones, and other compounds that are very similar to those found in the brain. Roughly half of all dopamine and 90 percent of the body's serotonin is produced by the ENS. Have you ever wondered why the antidepressant drugs known as selective serotonin reuptake inhibitors (SSRIs) often produce GI side effects? These drugs not only increase serotonin levels in the brain, but also in the gut, which can cause diarrhea and intestinal upset. It's long been observed that people with anxiety and depression often complain of GI problems, but research now suggests that it could be GI distress that triggers these mental states.

Although this may be hard to believe, I've witnessed the dramatic impact poor gut function can have on mental health in many patients over the years. One of my own family members, who lived with debilitating anxiety, experienced a dramatic improvement when she eliminated gluten from her diet. The point is that the brain and the ENS are in bidirectional communication. What affects one can impact the other.

The impact of stress on the gut may also be contributing to the enormous problem of obesity. Stress triggers the ENS to increase the production of ghrelin, a hormone that stimulates appetite. When we eat pleasurable foods (fatty and/or sugary foods), dopamine is released in the brain and in the gut, easing feelings of anxiety and depression. It's the brain in your gut that prods you to seek out those cookies when the boss is yelling at you! Chronic stress keeps ghrelin levels high, and the abundance of refined high-fat foods available 24/7 is a sure recipe for weight gain.

Make no mistake: Learning to manage your stress is a crucial part of improving your gut health, as well as enhancing your vitality overall. Much of what I wrote in *Life Is Your Best Medicine* was aimed at helping you learn to manage your stress by using meditation, movement, music, breath work, forgiveness, and wholesome foods. In addition to these strategies, many herbs can be of benefit.

Herbalists and physicians from ancient times have recognized the deep interconnection between the nervous and digestive systems. Many herbal formulations designed for easing depression or anxiety include herbs that also have beneficial effects upon the gut. Lemon balm, for instance, was once called the "gladdening" herb and has long been used to lift mood and ease anxiety. But this delightful member of the mint family has also been shown to ease colic, reduce intestinal gas and bloating, and improve irritable bowel syndrome. Many bitter herbs, which enhance digestion, also have calming effects on mood.

◗ The Gut Microbiome

It might surprise you to know that your intestines are composed of a vast, diverse, and enormously complex community of microbes, commonly referred to as your gut microbiota, and collectively referred to as the microbiome. More than 100 trillion microorganisms call the GI tract home. Microbes actually outnumber our own cells; in some respects, we're more bacteria than human. The microbiota are responsible for extracting and synthesizing vitamins and other nutrients from our food; regulating digestion, metabolism, and elimination; fine-tuning the immune system;

preventing the overgrowth of harmful bacteria; and maintaining the integrity and barrier function of the intestinal wall.

Over the millennia, the natural process of childbirth and breast-feeding has evolved to optimize our chance for survival. In the womb, the gut is sterile. The age of the infant at birth, and the method of delivery and early feeding all determine how the GI tract is colonized with bacteria. The intestinal tract of a full-term baby (37+ weeks) born vaginally is colonized by the mother's microbiota as the baby travels down the birth canal. Babies born prematurely, those exposed to perinatal antibiotics (for example, if the mom receives antibiotics during labor), or those delivered by cesarean section (C-section) do not acquire the same diverse and beneficial inoculation of microbes. And diversity is important for our health. Studies show that the microbiome of those with irritable bowel syndrome and atopic disease (asthma, allergies, and/or eczema) is much less diverse than healthy controls.

When babies are breast-fed, gut-friendly *Bifidobacteria* from the mother's nipples and milk ducts are ingested, and growth factors in the milk stimulate the development of a healthy intestinal mucosal lining. Breast milk also contains prebiotics, substances that encourage the growth of healthy microbiota, which may explain, in part, why breast-feeding has been associated with so many health benefits.

The microbiome plays a vital role in the development and maturation of the immune system, training it to recognize friend from foe. Studies show that children born by C-section are at greater risk for developing allergies, asthma, eczema, and celiac disease. In addition to our genetics, we're learning that an infant's diet and microbiota can also influence the development of autoimmune diseases, such as type 1 diabetes, multiple sclerosis, or inflammatory bowel disease.

The inappropriate prescribing of antibiotics, particularly in the first few years of life, as well as widespread use in livestock, is another big problem (see Chapter 2). Antibiotics destroy not only harmful pathogens but also friendly and healthy microbes. When levels of friendly microbiota are low, bacteria resistant to antibiotics thrive, making infections that much more difficult to treat in the future. Research shows that it can take up to four years for a microbiome to fully recover after antibiotic treatment. Antibiotics should only be taken when medically appropriate and necessary.

Given the profound impact our microbiome has on our overall health, major research efforts are under way to figure out the best ways to nourish and nurture this ecosystem. The good news is that there's a great deal you can do to improve your intestinal health, no matter how you were born or what your mother fed you. Science has shown that lifestyle and diet definitely affect the diversity of our gut microbiota. Removing any problematic foods in the diet is important. I cannot tell you how many people I've cared for whose migraines, IBS, allergies, and overall health dramatically improved once they eliminated dairy, gluten, and/or soy. Chronic stress suppresses the growth of beneficial bacteria, so learning to manage stress is vital. Adding more fermented and fiber-rich foods to the diet and taking a probiotic/prebiotic supplement can also do wonders.

◗ Making Friends With Healthy Microbes

Probiotics are living microorganisms that have a beneficial effect on intestinal health. The probiotic organisms most studied are *Lactobacillus, Bifidobacterium,* and *Streptococcus* bacteria, and the yeast *Saccharomyces boulardii.* These can be found in numerous dietary supplement products. Yogurt, kombucha tea, kefir, and other fermented foods are good sources of probiotics that can be easily added to your diet.

Prebiotics are a category of nondigestible nutritional compounds that promote the growth of beneficial gut bacteria, particularly *Bifidobacteria* and *Lactobacilli*. Prebiotic substances can be found in foods like garlic, onions, artichokes, asparagus, jicama, and burdock. Inulin, oligosaccharides, and fructooligosacchardes are examples of prebiotics found in dietary supplement products.

The term "synbiotic" is used to describe foods or products that contain both prebiotics and probiotics. Breast milk could be considered synbiotic as it contains oligosaccharides, and through the act of breast-feeding, babies also ingest *Bifidobacteria*.

I encourage all of my patients to include fermented foods and prebiotics in their diet. I recommend synbiotics for infants born by C-section, prematurely, or whose mothers received antibiotics during delivery. I also recommend them for those who have allergies, asthma, eczema, irritable bowel syndrome, constipation, recurrent vaginal infections, who travel internationally, or who've taken antibiotics. The simple truth is that I firmly believe most of us benefit from including these foods and/or supplements in our diet.

The research is constantly evolving, but based upon what we know today, the following strains I've listed have the best evidence for the following conditions:

Acute diarrhea. Some of the best evidence for the use of probiotics comes from studies of diarrhea in children, particularly diarrhea caused by rotavirus. The two most effective probiotics for diarrhea are *Lactobacillus rhamnosus GG (L. GG)* and *Saccharomyces boulardii (S. boulardii).*

Preventing diarrhea. Studies show that probiotics can also prevent diarrhea. Strains that have been studied include *Lactobacillus reuteri, L. GG, Lactobacillus casei,* and *S. boulardii.* For children in day care or for families with several young ones in the home, I strongly suggest giving one of these strains as a daily probiotic supplement.

Antibiotic-associated diarrhea. Studies in children and adults show that taking probiotics during antibiotic therapy lowers the risk of antibiotic-associated diarrhea, which occurs in 5 to 25 percent of people taking them. Take your probiotic 2 hours after each antibiotic dose and continue taking them for 4 to 8 weeks after finishing treatment to encourage the growth of healthy bacteria. *S. boulardii* and *L.* GG have the best evidence.

Traveler's diarrhea. Consider taking probiotics while traveling, especially in Mexico, South and Central America, Asia, and Africa. Taking a daily supplement with *S. boulardii* or *L.* GG can reduce your risk by about 40 percent.

Irritable bowel syndrome. Probiotics may help relieve some of the gas and bloating symptoms that accompany IBS. Look for products or yogurts that contain *Bifidobacterium infantis.*

Ulcerative colitis. Most physicians recommend VSL#3, a proprietary blend of four *Lactobacillus* strains, three strains of *Bifidobacterium,* and *Streptococcus salivarius* subsp. *thermophilus* that has been shown to improve symptoms and prevent relapse.

Atopic disease (AD). Preliminary studies show that when women take *L.* GG during the last month of pregnancy, it reduces the risk of AD in their children. If a baby is at high risk for AD (for instance, mom or dad has asthma, allergies, and/or eczema), studies show that when mom takes *L.* GG for the last four weeks of pregnancy and then both mom and baby take it for six months, it reduces the risk of AD by almost 50 percent. Some research shows that synbiotics can reduce the severity of AD in older children and adults.

Infant colic. Preliminary research has shown that probiotics, particularly *Lactobacillus reuteri,* can improve colic within about a week of treatment.

Vaginal infections. For women who have recurrent bacterial vaginosis or yeast infections, strains of *Lactobacillus rhamnosus* and *L. reuteri* have shown to help reduce recurrence when taken orally for several months.

General health maintenance. There has been little research in this area, but I generally recommend a synbiotic that includes a variety of *Lactobacillus* and *Bifidobacteria*.

When purchasing a probiotic supplement, look for a product that contains the correct strains. It's OK if there are additional *Lactobacilli* or *Bifidobacterium* in the product; just make sure the ones listed above are included. Follow the directions on the label. The dose needed for probiotics varies greatly depending on the strain and product. Dose also varies according to the probiotic strain, the product, and the intended use. In general, the research has found the following doses effective:

- *Lactobacillus rhamnosus* GG: 10 billion organisms once or twice a day
- *Lactobacillus reuteri:* 100 million organisms once or twice a day
- *Lactobacillus casei:* 1 to 10 billion organisms once a day
- *Saccharomyces boulardii:* 200 to 250 milligrams once or twice a day
- *Bifidobacterium infantis:* 100 million organisms once or twice a day

When purchasing yogurt, look for those that say "live and active cultures," and contain one or more of the strains listed previously.

Note: There have been a small number of cases of probiotics causing infection in people whose immune system was compromised. Although this has not been seen in healthy children or adults, I do not recommend giving probiotics to those who are critically ill or have intravenous catheters.

As you will see as you work your way through this section, if you are experiencing problems with irritable bowel syndrome, heartburn, constipation, diarrhea, eczema, food allergies, migraines, asthma, anxiety, or depression—getting your GI house in order is vitally important. We'll start with the esophagus/stomach and work our way down to the intestines.

▶ Digestive Discomforts: Easing Gas and Bloating

We've all had days when our bellies are so bloated that we cannot get our jeans to zip or we experience the embarrassment of gas loudly announcing itself. That's because, every day, the body produces small amounts of gas in our intestines. When we experience large or excessive amounts of gas, it's because the bacteria in our intestines are working overtime to break down only partially digested foods. Normally, stomach acid, bile, and pancreatic enzymes do an amazing job processing our food but if any of these are in short supply, it can lead to proliferation of bacteria in the small intestine and colon (see much more on this topic in the section on heartburn). Occasional gas and bloating is not a problem, but if you are dealing with gas, bloating, and indigestion on a regular basis, this is your body trying to tell you to get your digestive system in order. Here is some practical advice on things you can do at home.

Food Intolerances

Lactose intolerance occurs when you lack the lactase enzyme necessary for breaking down lactose, the natural sugar in dairy products. In this case, when the lactose reaches your colon, the bacteria go crazy, producing large quantities of hydrogen gas and causing abdominal cramping. With age, many of us lose our ability to digest lactose and experience more digestive troubles when we drink milk or eat too much cheese. If you think this might be a problem for you, eliminate all dairy products from your diet for two weeks and see if your symptoms disappear, or try taking lactase enzymes and see what happens.

Yogurt is often better tolerated than other forms of dairy because many contain *Streptococcus thermophilus* and/or *Lactobacillus delbrueckii* subsp. *bulgaricus,* which have been shown to reduce symptoms of lactose intolerance. That's why many people who cannot tolerate milk can eat yogurt containing these live cultures without difficulty.

In addition to dairy products, other foods are known to cause excessive gas:

- Asparagus, broccoli, Brussels sprouts, cabbage, and other vegetables
- Fructose, found in fruits and many, many foods as high-fructose corn syrup
- Foods high in soluble fiber, such as oat bran and fruits
- Whole grains, such as brown rice, oatmeal, and whole wheat
- Food high in starch like pasta, potatoes, and corn
- Sorbitol, an artificial sweetener

Keeping a food diary for a week can be particularly useful for identifying and then eliminating troublesome foods.

Digestive Enzymes

Digestive enzymes, available in supplements, can be helpful for persistent indigestion. Lactase pills or lactase-treated milk can dramatically improve your ability to digest dairy if you're not ready to give it up. Pancreatic enzymes can help you digest starches, fats, sugars, and proteins. They are extracted from both cattle and pigs, though most clinicians prefer the latter as they are more similar to enzymes our bodies produce naturally. If you prefer to get your enzymes from a nonanimal source, try supplements synthesized from microbial sources, such as lipases to digest fat from *Aspergillus oryzae* and lactase from *Kluyveromyces lactis*. Bromelain, extracted from pineapple stems, is helpful if you have a problem digesting protein. A blended enzyme product is usually most beneficial.

Generally, you'll take one to two capsules with meals, but follow the dosage recommendations on the supplement manufacturer's label.

Bitter Herbs

"Bitters" are herbs that, you guessed it, have a bitter taste. Our taste preferences, including an intense dislike for bitter, begin in our mother's womb. Ultrasounds show that, starting around the 16th week of pregnancy, babies strongly favor sweet-tasting substances. When something sweet is injected into the amniotic fluid, the baby sucks and swallows. When an innocuous bitter substance is injected, the baby closes its mouth tightly and ceases to swallow.

Most poisonous plants have a bitter acrid taste. Learning not to swallow bitter-tasting things likely afforded considerable protection for young infants who have a tendency to put everything in their mouths. Babies are also born with taste buds on the tongue, sides, and roof of their mouth, which intensifies all tastes. As we grow older, the taste buds disappear from everywhere but our tongue, making us less taste sensitive and able to enjoy a broader range of flavors such as bitter greens, coffee, and spicy foods.

Bitter herbs have been used to enhance digestion and elimination for thousands of years and may be one of the most important remedies in modern times if an optimally functioning digestive system is a key to good health. Bitter-taste receptors in the mouth stimulate the vagus nerve, which triggers a whole digestive chain reaction. This bitter stimulation increases salivation, stimulating the release of stomach acid and pancreatic enzymes, enhancing release of bile, and increasing gastric motility and lower esophageal sphincter tone. In other words: Bitters enhance almost every aspect of digestion. Bitter herbs are a foundational part of the vast majority of my treatment plans for patients, no matter what the primary problem.

It's essential that you actually experience the bitter taste to receive these wondrous benefits. Capsules and tablets are available, and although you can "dial back" the bitterness to increase palatability, it's important not to make them sweet. Herbs vary in their level of bitterness. One of my favorites is dandelion, whose genus name, *Taraxacum,* is actually an old word meaning "bitter herb." The greens and flowers can be eaten in salad or juiced, while the roots can be used fresh or dried as tea or tincture, or roasted and consumed as "poor man's" coffee. Studies have shown that dandelion root lowers inflammation in the body, nourishes the good bacteria in your colon, and is highly protective of your liver. Who knew? My mother gave me $1 for every grocery bag of dandelions I dug up in the garden! She thought they were pesky weeds! My Grandma Jo knew better, however. She cooked up dandelion greens the way most people cook spinach.

One of my favorite ways to take and administer bitters is in the form of a digestive aperitif. From the Latin *aperire,* meaning "to open," aperitifs are taken before meals to stimulate the appetite and prepare the GI tract. Angostura bitters are a classic example of a bitter aperitif. Angostura bitters are still readily available anywhere liquors are sold. Put 1 tablespoon in a glass of fizzy water and drink 15 to 20 minutes prior to a meal. It's pleasant tasting and highly effective for relieving gas, bloating, and heartburn. Or prepare your own Herbal Bitter Aperitif, following the recipe on pages 284–285. I've used an Herbal Bitter Aperitif in my practice for more than 30 years. A combination of bitters and carminatives, I've seen it work magic for those with poor digestive function.

Carminatives

Carminatives are herbs rich in volatile/aromatic oils that aid the body in expelling gas from the stomach and colon. Most culinary herbs and spices are carminatives. In addition to their amazing flavor, their digestive benefit was another reason they were commonly used in cooking. Some examples of carminatives include peppermint, fennel, anise, ginger, thyme, angelica, cardamom, cloves, and chamomile. The volatile oils, compounds like menthol that give peppermint its wonderful aroma, relax the muscles of the gastrointestinal tract, while increasing the flow of bile from the gallbladder, helping your body to more effectively digest fatty foods. This is why after-dinner mints and after-dinner liqueurs such as anisette, crème de menthe, and Sambuca are so popular.

If you have occasional indigestion, try drinking a cup of fennel, ginger, peppermint, or chamomile tea after dinner. It's best to avoid strong carminatives like peppermint or ginger if heartburn is a problem, as relaxing the lower esophageal sphincter can make reflux worse. If you experience heartburn frequently after a meal, along with gas and bloating, then take the Herbal Bitter Aperitif *before* meals.

Probiotics

Studies have shown that *Lactobacillus* species and *Bifidobacterium* strains can be very helpful for improving the gas and bloating that accompany irritable bowel syndrome (IBS). See "Making Friends With Healthy Microbes," pages 157–161.

|||||||||||||||||||||||||||||||||||||||||||||||||||||||||||||||||||||||||||||||||||||||||||||

☎ **When to Talk to Your Health Care Provider**
- If you experience a change in your digestion, including more gas and bloating, that doesn't resolve in a few weeks, even after trying some of these natural remedies

|||||||||||||||||||||||||||||||||||||||||||||||||||||||||||||||||||||||||||||||||||||||||||||

▶ Reflux Rears Up: Healing Heartburn

Many of us have had an episode of heartburn at some point in our lives, so I'm sure you're familiar with the burning sensation it creates. The pain may even radiate across your chest—a symptom often confused with a heart attack. Heartburn happens when the lower esophageal sphincter, a band of muscles responsible for preventing the backflow of contents from the stomach, fails to tighten. Delayed gastric emptying can also occur due to poor motility, a common problem as we age, but can also occur in any disorder that negatively impacts the nerves and/or muscles in the GI tract, such as diabetes, scleroderma, or hypothyroidism. Even chronic stress can alter gut motility. All of this can lead to stomach acids sloshing back up into the esophagus, irritating and inflaming its delicate lining.

Heartburn isn't a serious problem unless it starts occurring on a regular basis. When heartburn becomes chronic and/or intense, it's called gastroesophageal reflux disease (GERD). In conventional medicine, occasional heartburn is simply treated with over-the-counter antacids. For more persistent heartburn, proton pump inhibitor medications (PPIs), such as Nexium or Prilosec, are often tried. These drugs are highly effective at dialing down the acid-producing pumps in the stomach. You make less acid, thus less acid reflux. If these drugs don't relieve the symptoms, an endoscopy is performed, allowing a doctor to visualize the esophagus and stomach. This is important as a small number of people with persistent and/or severe GERD may over time develop scarring, narrowing, bleeding, and possibly even cancer in their esophagus if not properly treated.

Proton Pump Inhibitors: The Downside

According to the FDA, PPIs can make your magnesium levels plummet to dangerously low levels, causing problems ranging from muscle cramps to seizures and heart arrhythmias. When taken for more than a year, especially by people over the age of 50, PPIs reduce the absorption of calcium, iron, and vitamin B_{12}, and increase the risk for pneumonia and intestinal infections. These drugs are now required to carry a warning that they increase the risk for osteoporosis and fracture.

Because stomach acid is absolutely essential for destroying harmful microbes that may be present in your food, chronic use of these drugs also increases the risk of foodborne infections and pneumonia. Reducing stomach acid is thought to promote the growth of bacteria in our upper GI and respiratory tracts that are linked to pneumonia. A 2009 study published in the *Journal of the American Medical Association* concluded that roughly 33,000 deaths each year from pneumonia acquired while hospitalized are likely due to the PPIs patients are routinely put on when they are admitted.

If these facts aren't troubling enough, studies show that it can be really hard to get off these medications. Researchers at University of Copenhagen randomized 120 healthy volunteers who had no symptoms of acid reflux or any other gastrointestinal disorder into two groups for a 12-week study. One group received a placebo, and the other took 40 milligrams a day of esomeprazole (Nexium).

What happened was rather surprising: A whopping 44 percent of those who'd been taking the PPI developed significant acid reflux after going off them. These were people who didn't have heartburn before they took the drug.

There's a reason for this unlikely finding, though: After just a few weeks of taking the PPI, those acid-producing cells in your stomach multiply to try to overcome the drug's suppressant effect. When you stop the medication, you now have a whole army of cells pouring acid into your stomach. This phenomenon is called "rebound acid hypersecretion," and it's the main reason people end up staying on PPIs for so many years, even when they don't need them.

Bacterial Overgrowth

Although I don't object to the use of PPIs for more severe forms of GERD, the reality is that the problem for many people isn't too much stomach acid, but rather that they don't have enough. We need that low pH in our stomach to destroy bacteria and to digest our food. If we have insufficient stomach acid, bacteria are far more likely to proliferate in the small intestine. This condition, known as small intestinal bacterial overgrowth (SIBO), leads to symptoms such as excess gas, bloating, abdominal pain, heartburn, foul-smelling gas and stools, and diarrhea. SIBO can impair the absorption of important nutrients in the diet due to bacterial interference. This can lead to symptoms beyond the GI tract. A 2013 systematic review of 11 studies involving more than 3,000 patients published in *Clinical Gastroenterology and Hepatology* concluded that PPI use definitely increases the chances for SIBO.

A 54-year-old woman who had been on PPIs for six years came to see me because she'd been feeling increasingly depressed, tired, and irritable. She was past menopause and didn't feel it was a "hormonal issue." She couldn't identify any problems in her marriage or at work but she definitely didn't feel right. I did a number of laboratory tests and sent her for a hydrogen breath test to see if she had SIBO. She came back low in vitamins B_{12} and D, and magnesium, and she was positive for SIBO. I had her take 1,000 micrograms of vitamin B_{12}, 600 milligrams of magnesium, and 4,000 IU of vitamin D_3 every day for four months, and I treated her SIBO with Oregon grape root and probiotics. The difference in her mood and energy was dramatic. She told me how happy she was to "have her life back" but was also frustrated that the only treatment her primary care provider had offered her was an antidepressant prescription.

An Alternative Approach

For the vast majority of people with heartburn, weaning off PPIs can be done over a period of three to four months—time enough for your esophagus to heal and slow enough to prevent rebound hypersecretion. The following recommendations work really well for occasional heartburn, and I use this approach for tapering patients who are ready to come off PPIs. Talk to your health care provider to see if weaning is right for you.

Cool the Fire With Diet

Pay attention to any foods that you're eating that might be triggering your heartburn. The good news is that there are only a few foods that have been scientifically shown to trigger reflux: chocolate, deep-fried foods, coffee, alcohol, and peppermint or anything with peppermint oil. Chocolate and peppermint relax the lower esophageal sphincter (LES), allowing stomach contents to seep back into the esophagus. Fried foods take forever to digest, as do other fatty foods. The longer food sits in your stomach, the greater the risk for reflux. Triggers vary widely from person to person but you can try eliminating these to start with.

My main recommendation with regard to diet, however, is for people to go on a low-glycemic-load diet for 60 days. It can work magic for those with GERD. Patients who struggled with heartburn for years had it disappear in less than two weeks when they went on an Atkins/paleo/low-glycemic-load diet. Excessive carbohydrates in the diet can definitely increase gas and bloating, increasing abdominal pressure and forcing stomach contents back up in the esophagus.

||||||||||||||||||||||||||||||||||||||||||||||||||||||||||||||||||||||||||||||||||||||||||||||||||||||||||||

☎ Call Your Health Care Provider
- If your heartburn persists or worsens in spite of using natural home remedies or antacids
- If you have difficulty or pain when swallowing
- If you experience unintended weight loss
- If your stools are dark colored and/or tar-like

||||||||||||||||||||||||||||||||||||||||||||||||||||||||||||||||||||||||||||||||||||||||||||||||||||||||||||

Melatonin

You may know melatonin as a remedy for people who have a hard time falling asleep, but studies show it's also highly effective for relieving heartburn. Melatonin is a hormone secreted by the pineal gland, a small, flat, cone-shaped organ located in the lower-mid part of the brain. But specialized cells in the gastrointestinal tract also secrete melatonin, because one of its many jobs is to protect the esophageal lining from stomach acid. It does this in two ways: by tightening the LES, preventing the backflow of acid from the stomach, and by speeding the passage of food from the stomach into the small intestine. This makes it particularly important for those with poor gut motility caused by chronic stress, diabetes, or other things.

The incidence of heartburn has been on the rise over the past 20 years. Nearly 30 percent of all Americans complain of GERD. I wonder if this increase may be due, in part, to the fact that we watch television and work on computers late at night—both of which suppress the body's natural production of melatonin. The blue wavelengths from sunlight suppress melatonin, as does the blue light from televisions, lamps, computer screens, and many digital clocks. With melatonin in short supply, we may be losing its protective effect in the esophagus. We may be on to something here: Studies show that people with GERD or recurrent duodenal ulcers have lower melatonin levels than healthy individuals.

The studies evaluating the use of melatonin show that it works as well as Nexium in head-to-head double-blind studies after four weeks. Although the PPI and melatonin both alleviated heartburn, only the group receiving melatonin had a tightening of the LES. The dose of melatonin used in the clinical studies was 3 and 6 milligrams taken an hour or two before bedtime.

Melatonin has an excellent safety profile, far better than long-term PPIs, and should definitely be considered along with taking a bitter aperitif. If symptoms improve after 12 weeks, melatonin can be discontinued or decreased to 1 milligram.

Herbal Bitter Aperitif

I know many of you are thinking that taking bitters might make your heartburn worse, but I haven't found that to be the case. My favorite recipe (pages 284–285) contains dandelion, gentian, chamomile, fennel, and Oregon grape root. Dandelion contains inulin, a prebiotic to help balance out the microbiota. Dandelion and gentian are both bitters, which enhance and support healthy digestion and elimination. Oregon grape root is highly effective for eradicating SIBO when taken for six to eight weeks. Chamomile protects the gastric mucosa from the irritating effects of acid, and calms and quiets the enteric nervous system (ENS). Fennel is a carminative that helps relieve the symptoms of gas, bloating, and abdominal pain. Awesome, awesome medicine!

Herbal Demulcents for Occasional Heartburn

Herbs that soothe and protect irritated tissues are called "demulcents." These herbs are often rich in mucopolysaccharides, compounds that become "slimy" when they come in contact with water. They are ideal for relieving irritation of the mouth, throat, esophagus, stomach, and bowels. There are two you should always keep around the house:

- *Licorice* has been used for more than 3,000 years to soothe irritation and inflammation. It was widely used in Europe for the treatment of stomach ulcers during the 1940s and 1950s. However, roughly one in five people who took licorice for more than several months developed high blood pressure and had a dangerous drop in their potassium. Today, the compound that caused these problems can be removed, and the resulting product is sold as deglycyrrhizinated licorice (DGL). DGL can be safely taken long term. To use licorice to treat heartburn, chew 1 to 2 tablets for about 20 minutes before each meal. Original DGL tastes like black licorice, so if you're not a fan, choose chocolate or maple flavored.

- *Slippery elm bark* has been used for centuries to soothe sore throats, heartburn, and ulcers. As a matter of fact, the FDA still recognizes slippery elm bark as a safe and effective oral demulcent. Pick up some lozenges and keep them in your pantry for those times when you've overindulged on trigger foods. Unlike DGL, which is best taken before a meal for those prone to heartburn, slippery elm can be taken whenever needed. Chew 1 to 2 tablets.

Heartburn Relief Tea

Years ago, I got inventive and blended some gut-healing herbs— chamomile, a mild bitter herb with soothing, sedative effects; licorice, healing to the gut; and meadowsweet, with its antacid and anti-inflammatory attributes—and brewed them up as tea.

Meadowsweet was one of the plants used to synthesize aspirin. The word "aspirin" is derived from *Spiraea,* the old genus name

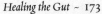
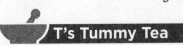

T's Tummy Tea

4 tablespoons chamomile flowers
2 tablespoons meadowsweet herb
2 tablespoons licorice root

Mix all the herbs together and put them in a glass jar. Screw on the lid, label the jar, and store it in your kitchen cupboard.

How to Use: Pour 1 cup near-boiling water over 1 heaping teaspoon of the herbal mixture. Steep for 10 minutes. Strain. Add honey if desired. Drink $\frac{1}{2}$ cup 1 to 2 times a day after the main meals of the day. This tea is gentle, tasty, safe, and effective when taken as directed.

Note: Although very unlikely to bother you at this dose, if you have high blood pressure, it's probably best to omit the licorice. If you are allergic to aspirin, substitute marshmallow leaf for meadowsweet.

---

for meadowsweet. But unlike aspirin, which can harm the stomach, meadowsweet is rich in mucilage, a gel-like substance that is healing to the stomach. Meadowsweet is very popular in Europe for treating heartburn. It has a pleasant flavor and aroma. Meadowsweet contains very small amounts of salicin, so to be on the safe side, avoid this herb if you're highly allergic to aspirin.

✚ Seek Medical Attention Now for Digestive Ailments

- If your heartburn is accompanied by pain in the neck, jaw, arms, or legs
- If you have shortness of breath, weakness, irregular pulse, or sweating
- If you have severe stomach pain
- If you have bloody vomit

▶ Infant Indigestion: Calming Colic

If you're a parent, I'm sure you can instantly sympathize when you hear a mother wearily say that she was up all night with her colicky baby. You know what it's like: Your otherwise happy, healthy baby drew up her knees, her face turned red, and she screamed for 20 to 30 minutes. How frustrating and stressful it can feel not to be able to soothe and calm your little one.

How do you know that your baby has colic? Well, the medical diagnosis is made when a healthy, well-fed baby between the ages of two weeks and four months cries and fusses more than three hours a day for three or more days in one week, for more than three weeks. Whew! Who's timing and counting?

Colic is a poorly understood condition in infants. There are lots of theories for what causes it, but no one really knows for sure. In some cases, it may be that babies are trying to learn how to balance their internal and external worlds. Remember, they lived in a watery womb for nine months where they had no hunger, thirst, wet diapers, bright lights, or chaos that often exists in busy families. Mom and baby are learning to get along, to communicate with one another, and to read each other's cues.

The lack of sleep that normally accompanies having a newborn in the house already makes moms and dads tired, but layering on hours of crying can stress out the most patient parent. If I'm describing you, I hope you have another caregiver who can help out with your newborn. This can be anyone who can take over for a couple hours each day—dad, an older sibling, a grandparent, extended family member, or friend. The bottom line is that it's OK to feel frazzled and frustrated. Colic will NOT last forever. In fact, it very rarely lasts beyond four months of age.

Carry and Quiet

Some babies are less fussy when carried in a sling or pack for several hours each day. The movement may help with digestion and mimic the sway of the mother when the babe was in the womb. I carried my infant son everywhere. He was strapped to my chest or back for hours at a time. We both loved it. He had an easy temperament and not much seemed to faze him. He could fall asleep anywhere.

However, when I tried doing the same with my infant daughter, the movement just stressed her out. The more I patted and bounced, the more she'd scream. She needed less stimulation, not more. And once she was in that overstimulated place, she found it very difficult to settle herself. I learned that she required longer periods of quiet with me, including low lights and low noise. She would nurse, quiet down, and sleep.

Finding that right balance of stimulation and quiet can be tricky. All babies are born with a relatively immature nervous system. And just as adults have different preferences and tolerance for noise and activity, babies do as well. This may be why some studies show that carrying babies improves colic, whereas others show no benefit. See what works best for your little one.

Diet for Mom and Baby

Some babies are sensitive to foods in the mother's diet or the type of formula they are drinking. Your baby may be intolerant of cow's milk proteins in your breast milk or to a cow's milk–based formula, for example. Excluding cow's milk from your diet if you're breast-feeding or switching to soy-based formula might help. Try this approach for seven to ten days to see if the colic improves. Adding lactase enzymes to formula can also be helpful. In one study, these enzymes reduced crying by 45 percent in colicky babies. Liquid lactase enzymes are available at grocery stores, health food stores, and pharmacies.

I generally recommend a hypoallergenic hydrolyzed whey protein formula for any baby who is not breast-fed and has a parent with a strong history of eczema, asthma, or allergies. Studies show that this type of formula not only improves colic, but it may help reduce the risk of the child developing eczema and asthma, as well.

And last but not least, if you're drinking fruit juice, try eliminating it for a week to see if the colic improves, or switch from apple to white grape juice. Colic in some babies appears to be caused by an inability to properly absorb sugars in apple juice.

Unfortunately, there isn't any easy way to predict which baby may be sensitive to what. It involves a lot of trial and error. Use your judgment and see if anything makes your baby's symptoms better.

Probiotics

Colic may affect babies who have an imbalance, or lack, of good bacteria in their intestines, according to a growing body of research. Studies have shown that babies with colic have far fewer of the beneficial bacteria, *Bifidobacteria* and *Lactobacilli*, in their stools compared to those who don't have colic.

The gastrointestinal (GI) tract of a baby in the womb is sterile. When a full-term baby travels through the vaginal birth canal, the GI tract is colonized with the mother's bacteria. Later, the mother's breast milk further populates the baby's GI tract with healthy bacteria.

A deficiency of these bacteria comes about when babies are born prematurely, by C-section, or if their mothers take antibiotics during labor. These situations interrupt the healthy colonization of bacteria that normally occurs with a full-term vaginal birth.

I see no downside and only a potential upside to giving a colicky baby a safe and high-quality probiotic. The two strains that have been studied for colic include *Lactobacillus reuteri* DSM 17938 and *Lactobacillus* GG. These can be found at natural foods grocers, health food stores, or online. They come in powder and liquids designed for infants. Use as directed.

Carminatives

As I mentioned in "Digestive Discomforts," page 165, carminatives are herbs that relieve intestinal gas and bloating. Chamomile, or *manzanilla* in Spanish, is used extensively by Latina mothers to soothe their babies. Lemon balm, like most members of the mint family, is a wonderful digestive aid, gently relaxing the gut muscles and easing gas, bloating, and indigestion, and it's suitable for the youngest children. In fact, a study of breast-fed babies with colic found that a combination of lemon balm, fennel, and chamomile decreased crying time by more than double compared to the babies receiving placebo over a period of one week!

Here are two simple recipes, an infusion and a glycerite, that I have used for many years in my practice. The tea is quick and easy to prepare; however, the Baby Tummy Soother is much easier to use, as you only have to give drops, not ounces, and the vegetable glycerin makes the herbs taste deliciously sweet.

Colic Relief Tea

1 tablespoon chamomile flowers
1 tablespoon lemon balm herb
1 tablespoon fennel seed

Mix the herbs together, place them in a jar with a tight-fitting lid, and label.

How to Use: Pour 1 cup near-boiling water over 1 teaspoon of the herb mixture. Steep for 5 minutes. Strain. Let cool. After feeding, offer 1 ounce of the tea. It's important to make sure the baby nurses or takes the bottle first, because those calories are needed. The tea comes at the end.

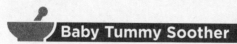

Baby Tummy Soother

10 grams chamomile flowers
10 grams lemon balm herb
5 grams fennel seed
140 milliliters vegetable glycerin
60 milliliters distilled/bottled water

Grind the herbs and put them in a jar. Cover with vegetable glycerin and water. Cover with a lid and let sit for 14 days, shaking daily. If the glycerite appears too thick, add another 20 milliliters vegetable glycerin and 5 milliliters water. After 2 weeks, strain the mixture through muslin cloth, pour into a dark bottle, and label. It will keep for 2 years.

How to Use: Give your baby 10 drops after each feeding, add it to the formula, or put it directly on your nipple before breast-feeding. Babies love the taste, and it is much easier to use than the tea. Make this ahead of time, so it's ready when you need it.

 Seek Medical Attention Now for an Infant With Colic

- If your baby is fussy and refuses to nurse or take a bottle for more than six hours
- If your baby has a fever, vomiting, or bloody stools

◐ Nausea and Vomiting: Settle Your Stomach Naturally

When you feel queasy and your stomach starts doing somersaults, it can be unsettling and worrisome. And rightfully so! This ancient and highly protective response is designed to defend the body against poisons. Messages are sent from the gut, the inner ear, and/or the chemoreceptor trigger zone (CTZ) to the vomiting center in your brain, which interprets the information and determines whether or not vomiting should be initiated. Nausea, that sick feeling you get before vomiting, is intended to prevent you from eating or drinking, in case something is wrong with the food or beverage. The inner ear and CTZ are specifically designed to detect toxins in the blood. This is why chemotherapy drugs and excessive alcohol intake, for example, cause nausea and vomiting—the body perceives them as poisons and is attempting to expel them.

Sometimes the message gets confused. For instance, when fluids in the ear are thrown about in different directions, such as when riding on a merry-go-round or riding in a boat, the brain thinks there's something wrong. Interestingly, the Latin root word for nausea actually means "seasickness"!

Although we're not sure exactly what causes morning sickness in pregnancy, many scientists believe it's due to shifting hormone levels. However, biologists—noting that pregnant women are more sensitive to smells and tastes—hypothesize that morning sickness is part of a heightened response designed to protect the baby from any toxins or poisons the mother might ingest.

So although unpleasant, the ability to vomit is a highly important part of our body's defense system. The "stomach flu," or gastroenteritis, affects more than 20 million Americans every year. These 24- to 48-hour "bugs" are usually caused by viral infections, though they can be caused by bacteria, parasites, or protozoa, and have nothing to do with influenza. A flu shot won't protect you! Rotavirus is the most common cause of gastroenteritis in children, whereas noroviruses primarily affect teens and adults. Washing your hands is the best means of protection because these viruses spread via the fecal-oral route (yes, I know, very gross). You can pick them up from a doorknob or by eating food prepared by cooks who didn't wash their hands after using the restroom. Gastroenteritis often causes both vomiting and diarrhea. In most cases, you don't want to suppress this forceful evacuation; it's helping you clear the infection or tainted food. (See the section on diarrhea for more information.)

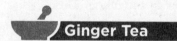

Ginger Tea

Pour 1 cup near-boiling water over ¼ teaspoon dried powdered ginger. Let it steep for 10 minutes. Carefully pour off the liquid, leaving the powder settled in the bottom of the cup. If desired, add a small amount of honey.

For morning sickness: Drink ¼ cup of ginger tea 3 to 4 times a day. It is safe to use in pregnancy, but do not exceed this amount of tea. If taking capsules, do not take more than 1,000 milligrams of dried ginger a day. (For more tips on morning sickness, see the sections on moms-to-be).

For motion sickness: Drink ½ cup of ginger tea an hour prior to travel. Then drink ¼ cup every 1 to 2 hours, as needed. Ginger capsules may be more convenient when traveling. Take 500 milligrams every 4 hours and up to 2,000 milligrams a day.

For chemotherapy-associated nausea: Drink ¼ cup 4 times a day for 3 days BEFORE you go in for treatment, then again the day of and day after treatment. Ginger must be taken before treatment for maximum benefit. If taking capsules, take 500 milligrams every 4 to 6 hours, up to 2,000 milligrams a day. Ginger will not interfere with your medications. I also highly recommend the book *One Bite at a Time* by Rebecca Katz for practical and insightful tips on eating while undergoing chemo treatments. If you need something stronger than ginger and acupuncture, ask your doctor to give you a prescription drug like ondansetron (Zofran).

However, when you're going to go on a cruise or are undergoing chemotherapy treatments, consider using some preventive strategies, like ginger tea and acupressure, to keep the queasiness at bay.

Ginger for Prevention

Ginger is a very effective antiemetic. Although commonly referred to as "ginger *root*," it is actually a rhizome, or underground stem. Plenty of science supports ginger as a terrific stomach settler. Ginger is a popular home remedy for indigestion and has been clinically studied and found effective for relieving morning sickness, motion sickness, and chemotherapy-induced nausea and vomiting. Dried ginger is a more potent antiemetic than fresh ginger, although both can ease nausea.

Ginger Candy or Snaps

If you don't like the taste of ginger tea, candied ginger works really well. Just suck on it as you would a piece of hard candy. I've also had patients swear by old-fashioned ginger snap cookies.

Acupressure to the Rescue

Used by the Chinese for more than 5,000 years, acupressure, the pressure of hands and fingers on the body, has been used to promote health and alleviate pain.

Studies have shown that applying pressure to a particular point on the inside of your forearm, just above the wrist, can ease nausea and vomiting from a number of causes. You can locate this point, called pericardium 6 (P6), in the following manner:

- Turn your hand so that your palm is facing up.

- Move your other hand down your forearm about two inches away from the crease in your wrist.
- Poke gently between the tendons until you find a spot that's a little tender.

That's it! Now you just need to apply steady, firm pressure on the spot for about ten minutes. This can be repeated every hour, as needed. I think everyone should be familiar with this acupressure point. You can do it on yourself or perform it on others. There are no side effects. I've seen it work many times for easing morning sickness and motion sickness.

Acupuncture, the insertion of very thin needles into specific areas of the body, is more effective than acupressure for those with more severe morning sickness or who are undergoing che-motherapy. To find a licensed practitioner in your area, go to the National Certification Commission for Acupuncture and Oriental Medicine website at *www.nccaom.org*.

What to Do When You Vomit

If you're throwing up, you should keep a few things in mind. Although most people kneel in front of the toilet, that's not the best position, especially for a child. You want your head to be lower than your stomach to prevent aspirating the vomit into your lungs. Stay standing up, put your hands on the toilet seat for support, and then bend over so that your face is just four to six inches above the toilet opening.

Your natural inclination is going to be to drink something to get rid of the bad taste in your mouth. But don't rush this! You'll just make yourself vomit again! It's OK to rinse your mouth with water or suck on some ice chips (peppermint ice chips are great), but it's important to let your stomach stop revolting before try-ing to fill it with liquid. Do NOT attempt to drink anything for 2 hours after throwing up. After 2 hours, sip 2 to 3 ounces of fluid (such as tea, sports drinks, carbonated drink, or water) every 10 to 15 minutes for 3 to 4 hours. If you vomit again, start this process all over.

Four hours or so after your last episode of vomiting, you can slowly begin to eat easily digested foods, such as crackers and toast. If you keep these down, try rice, bananas, applesauce, or soup, but be careful not to eat anything too spicy or fatty too soon.

Peppermint Ice Cubes

Peppermint is an old and trusted remedy, especially as a tea, for easing nausea, vomiting, and diarrhea. But over the years, I've found that the smell and the taste of hot tea can be overwhelming for some folks. A wonderful alternative is peppermint ice chips. They go down easy, work amazingly well, and taste delicious. Make them ahead of time and keep them on hand in your freezer.

How to Use: Put 4 to 5 ice cubes in a blender to break them into pieces. Then just suck on them slowly or use a spoon and let a small amount melt in your mouth. Peppermint ice cubes help lower fever, ease nausea, and leave your mouth and throat feeling cool and fresh. I have used these for my patients, kids, and myself over the years. You can safely consume them during pregnancy, and they are perfectly safe for children.

German Chamomile

Chamomile is also a wonderful and soothing herb if you feel sick to your stomach, especially when the nausea is accompanied by diarrhea. Chamomile soothes, protects, and eases spasms in the stomach and intestines. It's also a nice calmative, making you feel a little better when you're feeling bad.

Chamomile is very safe and is my herb of choice when looking for something to settle an infant's upset tummy. I remember the

Chamomile Infusion

2 teaspoons German chamomile flowers
1 cup water

Put the chamomile flowers in a mug and pour freshly boiled water over the herb. Let it steep 3 to 5 minutes. Strain the liquid through a tea strainer.

How to Use: Drink 1 to 2 cups to settle the stomach, to soothe the nerves, or just to make the world feel a little less chaotic. If desired, add a dab of honey and/or lemon.

Note: You may have heard that some people with severe ragweed allergies may also have allergies to chamomile. Although this can occur, it is actually quite rare.

---

time my oldest came down with a "stomach bug," when he was about 14 months old. I gave him shaved chamomile ice cubes to suck on. I drank a couple cups of chamomile tea myself, because neither one of us was getting any sleep! Chamomile is an herbal lullaby—and every mother's ally.

Abdominal Massage

One of my most tender memories of childhood was when I was about seven years old and staying at my Grandma Jessie's house. In the middle of the night, she found me throwing up in the bathroom. She kneeled beside me, pulled my hair away from my face, and gently rubbed my back. After I had finished vomiting, Grandma Jessie went into the kitchen and got a washcloth, a towel, and a bowl. We went back to my room, and she put the cool washcloth on my head. She placed the bowl and towel on the nightstand in case I needed it. Then she began to rub my belly in little circles, working her way around my abdomen in a clockwise motion. She spoke softly and told me that her mother used to rub her tummy like this when she was sick as a little girl. It felt so good. Everything felt good: her hands, her voice, the feeling of being cared for and loved. That night, I learned the powerful medicine that is *tender loving care.*

You will find more detailed instructions for abdominal massage in the section on constipation, page 196. This should be a light and gentle massage. If the massage causes pain, stop. This could indicate that something more serious is going on, such as appendicitis.

✚ Seek Medical Attention Now for Nausea or Vomiting

- If you have vomited for longer than 48 hours (for adults and children), or 12 hours for children under the age of a year
- If you are unable to keep any liquids down after 12 hours
- If there is bloody vomit
- If you experience severe or progressively worsening abdominal pain
- If you have chest pain
- If you suffer from a headache, stiff neck, and fever
- If you show signs of dehydration, such as dry mouth, no tears, infrequent urination, or dark urine
- Infants under the age of two months of age who are vomiting (not typical spit-up) should be quickly evaluated by a health care practitioner.

▶ Gut Check: Diarrhea

Most of us have battled diarrhea at some point. Those loose, watery stools are usually caused by infections that don't last long, and are more of a nuisance than a danger for most healthy people. Gastroenteritis, an inflammation/infection of the GI tract, generally lasts one to three days, and can be easily managed by staying hydrated while it "runs" its course. However, diarrhea can be dangerous for the very young, the very old, and those with serious underlying disease. Globally, 90 percent of deaths from diarrheal diseases are due to unsafe water and sanitation, and occur in children under five years of age. Even in the United States, diarrhea accounts for more than 8 million visits to the doctor's office and 250,000 hospitalizations annually. In developed nations, viral infections are the most common cause of acute diarrhea, followed by bacterial infections, food poisoning (particularly seafood), and infections by parasites and protozoa.

Staying Hydrated

You might be thinking that staying hydrated sounds pretty straightforward, but when I was doing my internship at the University of New Mexico hospital, our team admitted so many young children for dehydration due to rotavirus that the hospital ran out of beds and had to divert patients to other area hospitals. Learning how to prevent dehydration is important, because almost every child in the United States by the age of five will be infected with the rotavirus, the most common cause of severe diarrhea among infants and young children. Vomiting is often the first symptom of this virus, followed by watery diarrhea and fever. Rotavirus is highly contagious and spreads quickly. One gram (about the size of a cherry) of stool can contain more than 10 trillion infectious particles, and it takes fewer than 100 of those particles to pass the infection to someone else. These infectious particles can survive for several days on doorknobs, sink handles, and toys, which is why frequent hand-washing is so important for children and their caregivers.

Preventing dehydration is the number one priority, and the kind of fluid you use is important. In infectious diarrhea, the lining of the intestine becomes inflamed, impairing its ability to absorb water. When you drink water, it travels down through the intestines, unabsorbed, resulting in even more diarrhea. If you put salt in the water, essentially the same thing happens.

Roughly 40 years ago, researchers discovered that the absorption of salt is linked to glucose, which means that by simply adding sugar, the salt and water are absorbed and the body can be rehydrated. This discovery led to the development of sports drinks, such as Gatorade, and children's oral rehydration solutions, like Pedialyte. (Babies should not be given sports drinks for rehydration because they do not contain the correct ratio of ingredients.)

Keeping a bottle of sports drink on hand, or if you have small children, a bottle of Pedialyte can sure come in handy when you need it! Of course, with some basic kitchen ingredients, you can easily make your own oral rehydration solution.

The World Health Organization, UNICEF, the Centers for Disease Control, and pediatric/medical societies around the

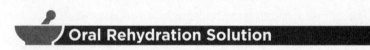

Oral Rehydration Solution

$4\frac{1}{2}$ cups (1 liter) clean water
$\frac{1}{2}$ teaspoon salt
6 level teaspoons sugar

Combine all ingredients. Stir until the sugar and salt have dissolved. You can add $\frac{1}{2}$ cup orange juice to improve the flavor and provide roughly 260 milligrams of potassium. Or substitute 2 teaspoons sugar with 2 teaspoons molasses, which provides roughly 350 milligrams of potassium. Make fresh daily.

How to Use: Give your infant or young child $\frac{1}{2}$ cup or more after every stool. For an older child or adult, give 1 cup or more after every stool.

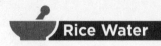

Rice Water

1 cup rice
4 cups water

Put 1 cup rice in 4 cups water, and bring to a boil. Cover, turn down heat, and simmer for 20 minutes. Strain the milky water.

How to Use: Drink throughout the day. Not only is this good for humans, it is one of the best things you can do for dogs with diarrhea. You can add $\frac{1}{2}$ cup chicken broth to increase their desire to drink it.

---

world advocate the use of this simple rehydration solution, which costs only pennies to make and has saved the lives of millions of children around the world.

In *addition* to these fluids, anyone suffering from diarrhea should also drink generous amounts of water, rice water, diluted fruit juice (one part juice to three parts water), and/or herbal teas. Rice water is excellent for hydrating the body and slowing diarrhea.

What to Eat When Treating Diarrhea

If your newborn has diarrhea, continue breast-feeding or giving formula. Studies show that most infants can tolerate lactose formulas without worsening diarrhea. For older children and adults, I often recommend avoiding dairy products for a few weeks, with the exception of probiotic-rich yogurt, because diarrhea can cause temporary lactose intolerance.

Another diet "cure" is the BRAT diet (bananas, rice, applesauce, and toast). Mashed bananas are high in potassium, and the pectin in bananas and applesauce help firm up stools. To ease nausea and intestinal cramping, add ¼ teaspoon ground cinnamon. As for white rice (served plain) and toast, they're both easy to digest. Most adults and older children can otherwise resume their normal diet within a couple days, but it's sensible to initially avoid spicy, greasy, and fatty foods.

||||||||||||||||||||||||||||||||||||||||||||||||||||||||||||||||||||||||||||||||||||||||||||||||||||

☎ Call Your Health Care Provider
- If an infant or child with diarrhea isn't better in 24 hours
- If an adult with diarrhea isn't better in 3 days
- If you've been traveling or possibly drinking contaminated water

||||||||||||||||||||||||||||||||||||||||||||||||||||||||||||||||||||||||||||||||||||||||||||||||||||

Garlic

Garlic is a wonderful food for helping your body fight off diarrhea. Garlic can kill many of the bacteria that cause gastroenteritis and diarrhea. Louis Pasteur was the first to scientifically document its potent effect against bacteria and fungus, and Dr. Albert Schweitzer used garlic extensively to treat dysentery and cholera while working as a missionary in Africa. Garlic honey is an easy and effective way to take garlic, as raw garlic can sometimes be too much for a sensitive tummy.

Probiotics

As I discussed in the introduction to this chapter, probiotics are vitally important for the health and integrity of the GI tract. Some of the best evidence for probiotics comes from research of children with diarrhea, particularly diarrhea caused by rotavirus. Probiotics, particularly *Lactobacilllus reuteri* and *Saccharomyces boulardii,* shorten the duration and reduce the severity of diarrhea. And if one person in the house has come down with gastroenteritis, then make sure you give everyone else in the household probiotics as well. For children in day care, families with several young ones in the home, or elders in nursing home facilities, I strongly suggest giving one of these strains as a daily probiotic supplement.

R̲X̲ PRESCRIPTION FROM DR. LOW DOG
Peppermint for IBS

Science has shown that enteric-coated peppermint oil capsules are more effective than conventional treatments for relieving irritable bowel syndrome (IBS), particularly when diarrhea is prominent. The enteric coating allows more peppermint oil to reach the intestine where it reduces bloating and cramping. The dose is 0.2 milliliter peppermint oil capsules taken 15 to 20 minutes before meals.

German Chamomile

A number of herbs are beneficial for diarrhea: peppermint, catmint (catnip), and ginger. But my hands-down go-to herb in these cases is German chamomile, as it eases the cramping that accompanies diarrhea and quiets intestinal inflammation. Chamomile tastes pleasant and can be given to babies and elders.

How to Use: Chamomile infusion: For babies under the age of 1, offer 1 ounce *after* nursing or formula feeding. For children 1 to 3 years of age: 2 ounces 4 to 6 times a day. Over 4 years of age: Drink as often as desired through the day.

German Chamomile Glycerite OR Baby Tummy Soother (pages 287 or 178):

15–60 pounds: 1 drop per pound of body weight 3 times a day

60–100 pounds: 1 teaspoon 3 times a day

Teens and adults: 1 tablespoon 3 times a day

Note: Chamomile is extremely safe. However, rare reports of allergic reactions have been reported in those with severe allergies to plants in the daisy family.

Nature's Antimicrobials

Nature has provided a number of powerful anti-infective herbs. The herbs I've relied on for treating infectious diarrhea are those that contain berberine, a bitter, yellow alkaloid found in goldenseal, barberry, Oregon grape root, and goldthread. Berberine-rich herbs have been extensively used in traditional medicine to treat diarrhea and dysentery. Modern science has confirmed that berberine is highly active against *Escherichia coli, Giardia lamblia,* and *Entamoeba histolytica,* three organisms that cause infectious diarrhea. Berberine inhibits the ability of *E. coli* to adhere to bladder and intestinal mucosa, reducing its ability to cause infection, and inhibits the growth of protozoa, such as *Giardia* and *Entamoeba.* These herbs also act as astringents, reducing inflammation in the intestinal tract and helping to prevent dehydration.

I cared for one patient who'd developed persistent diarrhea after becoming infected with *Entamoeba histolytica* while traveling in India. He'd been treated with multiple rounds of metronidazole, the drug of choice for this infection, but his stool cultures showed he still had the infection. I gave him barberry root bark tincture for three weeks. His diarrhea cleared and his stool culture came back negative. I've also used these herbs to treat stool-positive *Giardia,* a common parasite found in many rivers and streams, in both humans and dogs. I believe it will become increasingly important to understand how and when to use natural antimicrobial plants, given the growing problem of antibiotic resistance, as well as for those of us who live, camp, or backpack in remote areas where we have limited access to antimicrobial drugs.

Barberry or Oregon Grape Root

Prepare the Barberry or Oregon Grape Root Tincture in "The Eighteen Essentials" (page 281) or the Barberry Glycerite shown here.

How to Use: Adults should take 3 milliliters of the tincture 3 to 4 times a day for 2 to 3 weeks. Pets and children should use barberry glycerite.

WARNING: Berberine-containing herbs should not be used during pregnancy or while breast-feeding.

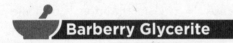

Barberry Glycerite

25 grams barberry root bark, dried
90 milliliters vegetable glycerin
35 milliliters water

Grind barberry root bark to a coarse powder and put in a glass jar. Add vegetable glycerin and water. Stir with a spoon. If you need more liquid, add an additional 20 milliliters glycerin and 5 milliliters water. Replace the lid. Shake daily for 2 to 4 weeks. Pour the contents of the jar into fine cheesecloth and strain, squeezing firmly to remove all liquid. Compost the herbs. Pour the liquid into a dark glass bottle and label. The glycerite will keep for 2 years.

How to Use:
15 to 25 pounds: 1 milliliter 3 times a day
26 to 40 pounds: 1.5 milliliters 3 times a day
41 to 60 pounds: 2 milliliters 3 times a day
61 to 90 pounds: 3 milliliters 3 times a day
Over 90 pounds: 3 to 5 milliliters 3 times a day

If you have children or pets in the house, or adults who don't like or cannot tolerate alcohol, you should consider keeping some barberry glycerite around the house. Even though the kids are grown, I keep the glycerite around the house to use with the dogs and cats when they come down with diarrhea.

Seek Medical Attention Now for Diarrhea

Seek care immediately if diarrhea is accompanied by:
- Severe abdominal pain
- Blood in stool
- Fever in an infant under three months of age
- A fever of 103°F or higher in child or adult
- Dry mouth or crying without tears (dehydration)
- Skin that doesn't flatten when pinched and released (dehydration)

◑ Constipation: Cures That Will Move You

Constipation isn't the sexiest condition to talk about but approximately 2.5 million Americans consult a doctor for this problem. And my practice has been no exception. Constipation is medically defined as having a bowel movement fewer than three times a week. Although not usually life threatening, the pain, bloating, fullness, and straining associated with constipation can make you beg for one thing—relief. And that often means laxatives. Every year, Americans spend $725 million on over-the-counter laxatives! If you're among those who suffer with constipation, take heart: You can treat it effectively with diet, lifestyle, and a few gentle, easy-to-make home preparations.

For background, let's review what normally happens after your food has been digested and enters your colon, or large intestine. As the food travels through your colon, water is absorbed back into your body, and the waste products, or stool, are pushed toward the rectum by strong muscle contractions. By the time the stool reaches your rectum, it is solid, because most of the water has been absorbed. Constipation occurs when either too much water is absorbed and/or the muscle contractions are slow or sluggish.

Ignoring the urge to have a bowel movement is a big reason many people struggle with constipation. I cannot tell you how many times people have told me that they've been embarrassed to have a BM at the office because they don't want anyone to hear them in the next stall. Children learn to ignore the call when they're not allowed to use the restroom during class, and they're often too distracted and busy playing at recess to think about it. Always heed the call of nature. If you don't like using a public restroom, allow time to use the bathroom at home every morning after breakfast.

Unhealthy dietary habits are another common cause. I'm mainly talking about having too little liquid and/or fiber in your diet. Constipation is often the result of dehydration, so drinking water keeps everything moving. You definitely know you need to drink more fluids when the stool is hard and difficult to pass. Caffeinated and alcoholic drinks don't count, either. They act like diuretics, emptying your body of water and causing further dehydration.

As for fiber, most of us fall far short of the 30 grams recommended by the American Dietetic Association, in no small part because the natural fibers have been removed from refined foods Americans love to eat. Provided you drink enough water daily, fiber eases constipation by making your stool softer and bulkier. High-fiber foods include beans, bran cereals, whole grains, fresh fruits, and vegetables.

In many instances, constipation arises from the modern couch-potato lifestyle lacking in regular exercise. Physical inactivity can definitely lead to lazy and sluggish bowels.

Certain medical conditions can trigger constipation, too. Any neurological disorder that interferes with nerve impulses in your colon can slow down muscle contractions. Constipation is a common symptom of hypothyroidism, a condition in which the thyroid gland does not make enough thyroid hormone. People suffering from irritable bowel syndrome with predominantly constipation also have pain and bloating as part of their symptoms.

Paradoxically, taking stimulant laxatives (like senna or cascara sagrada) can cause constipation, as well. Laxatives can become habit-forming, making it hard to have a bowel movement without them. And up to 150 prescription medications are known to cause constipation. Make sure to talk to your doctor or pharmacist for advice if either of these situations applies to you.

You can take a number of lifestyle measures, along with natural remedies, to alleviate constipation without resorting to over-the-counter drug treatments.

Lifestyle Changes to Fend Off Constipation

- Here's an easy way to form a good water-drinking habit. Each morning, fill a quart container with water and add one or more of the following: sliced cucumber, lemon, oranges, strawberries, or one to two peppermint ice cubes. Sip from this quart throughout the day, making sure you finish it before dinner. It is easy to miscalculate the amount of water you are drinking. One quart provides four cups and should be the *minimum* you are drinking if you have constipation.
- Walk for at least 30 minutes every day or do more vigorous exercise if you're up for it. Physical activity stimulates muscle contractions in the colon.
- Eat more vegetables and fruits—at least five servings or more a day. Dark green veggies such as kale, spinach, turnip greens, and others are really important because they're loaded with constipation-fighting magnesium as well as fiber.

||||||||||||||||||||||||||||||||||||||||||||||||||||||||||||||||||||||||||||||||||||||||||||

☎ Call Your Health Care Provider
- If you have blood in your stool, or dark tar-like stools
- If you have pain during or after bowel movements
- If you have constipation accompanied by unexplained weight loss
- If you notice a change in bowel habits, particularly after age 50

||||||||||||||||||||||||||||||||||||||||||||||||||||||||||||||||||||||||||||||||||||||||||||

Abdominal Massage

When I went to massage school and learned how to perform abdominal massage, I understood just how powerful it could be for relieving constipation and indigestion. You can perform massage on yourself, and I strongly encourage you to do it morning and night for five minutes. It will definitely improve your situation. Here's how to do it:

1. Lie down in a comfortable place, place a pillow underneath your knees, and put a little lotion or massage oil (such as my Belly Massage Oil) on your hands.
2. Beginning in your lower right pelvic area, gently apply pressure and massage in small circles, slowly moving upward toward your rib cage.
3. When you get to the right side of your rib cage, gently but firmly massage toward the outer edge of your left rib cage.
4. Work your way down the left side of your torso toward your groin area.
5. As you massage, you may find some areas that are tender when you apply pressure. Spend a little more time in those areas, massaging gently but firmly. Over time, these areas will become less tender, and your constipation will improve.
6. Do this morning and night, gradually increasing the pressure.

Note: If the pain in your abdomen is severe or doesn't improve, discontinue massage and see your health care provider. And do not do deep massage on your tummy if you're pregnant.

Belly Massage Oil

4 tablespoons (2 ounces) olive, grape seed, or sesame oil
12 drops peppermint or lavender essential oil

Mix together and put in a dark colored bottle.

Magical Magnesium: A Natural Laxative

With all the focus on calcium, this amazing mineral has been sadly overlooked. Magnesium helps to increase insulin sensitivity and blood sugar control, maintain a normal heart rhythm and blood pressure, and prevent migraine headaches and is actively involved in the contraction/relaxation of muscles.

In addition to all the health benefits associated with magnesium, this mineral is an excellent and reliable stool softener and laxative that is not habit-forming. Whenever someone is struggling with chronic constipation, I recommend 400 to 600 milligrams of chelated magnesium (such as citrate, malate, or glycinate) taken at bedtime. It never fails.

Note: This amount of magnesium is considered to be quite safe. However, if you have poor kidney function, do not take supplemental magnesium without talking to your health care provider first.

Just the Flax, Please!

Flax *(Linum usitatissimum)* was one of the earliest cultivated crops in the Fertile Crescent, in approximately 7000 B.C. It was primarily used for the production of linen, hence the genus name *Linum,* from the Greek meaning "net" or "cloth." For centuries, flax was spun into threads to produce linen cloth.

Flaxseeds are also known by the common name, linseed. The painter Jan van Eyck is credited with having created a varnish using linseed and other oils in the 1400s. Modern linseed oil is still made from flaxseed, but is boiled and contains other ingredients that make it unsuitable for human ingestion.

Today, flaxseeds make a wonderful addition to the diet, providing an excellent source of omega-3 fatty acids, lignans, and both soluble and insoluble fiber. Both the fiber and omega-3 fatty acids make it a heart-friendly food choice, and flax is virtually unrivaled when it comes to dietary lignans, natural antioxidants that help protect cells from damage and may give the body an edge against breast and prostate cancer. Flaxseeds have up to 700 times more lignans than legumes and whole grains.

Flaxseeds are golden or brown; both contain similar levels of healthy components, so either is fine. Whole and ground flax-seeds have the same nutritional value, but ground flaxseed is

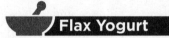

Flax Yogurt

1 tablespoon flaxseeds, ground
1 cup (8 ounces) live-culture Greek-style yogurt
Handful of fresh fruit in season, washed
Pinch of cinnamon

Use a coffee grinder to grind the flaxseeds into a powder and mix into the yogurt. Pour the yogurt over fresh fruit.

How to Use: Eat 1 cup every day to increase dietary fiber and healthy probiotics, and to improve regularity.

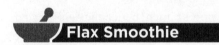

Flax Smoothie

1 cup almond milk
1 to 2 tablespoons flaxseeds, ground
$\frac{1}{2}$ cup raspberries, strawberries, or blackberries
1 tablespoon almond butter

Grind the flaxseeds in a coffee grinder. Put all the ingredients into a blender and blend on high for 30 to 45 seconds.

How to Use: Pour into a glass and enjoy. It's high in fiber and protein and low in calories—delicious! You can substitute dairy, soy, or coconut milk for the almond milk.

more easily digested. Buy whole flaxseeds and either grind them as you go, or grind and store them in an airtight container in your refrigerator for up to 60 days. I often incorporate flaxseeds in cooking, substituting them for some of the oil and/or eggs in a recipe. One tablespoon of flaxseeds contains approximately 5 grams of fiber. The equivalents work like this:

Egg substitute: Add 1 tablespoon ground flaxseed to 3 tablespoons water. Let this mixture sit for 2 minutes, and you've created the equivalent of one egg. I love this substitute when a recipe calls for eggs, and I'm out or I just want to pump up the fiber in the dish.

Oil substitute: Use 1 cup ground flaxseed to replace ⅓ cup oil. This substitution works because of the natural oils already present in freshly ground flaxseed. You'll increase the fiber and omega-3 content of your dish, plus obtain the benefit of those powerful lignans. Note: Your baked goods will brown a little faster with this substitution.

Herbal Laxatives

I've made my share of herbal laxative teas for patients over the years. My favorite herbs include senna, a well-known and established laxative; licorice, an excellent stool softener; and dandelion root, a mild bitter that promotes the release of bile, a natural laxative. I include ginger, fennel, and/or cardamom to prevent the intestinal cramping that often occurs with any laxative use.

 Seek Medical Attention Now for Constipation

- If you have a fever with severe abdominal pain
- If you have severe abdominal pain

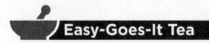

Easy-Goes-It Tea

4 teaspoons dandelion root
4 teaspoons senna leaves
2 teaspoons licorice root
2 teaspoons fennel seed
1 teaspoon ginger rhizome/root, cut (not powder)

Blend the herbs together and store them in a jar. This herbal mixture will stay good for approximately 2 years if kept in an airtight container and stored in a cool, dark cupboard. This tea is only for occasional use as a laxative and may be taken safely for 5 to 7 days.

How to Use: Place 2 teaspoons herbal mixture in 12 ounces cool water and bring to a boil. Cover, turn off heat, and steep for 20 minutes. Strain. Store in the refrigerator and drink cold or at room temperature. Take $\frac{1}{4}$ cup in the morning and night. You can increase your dosage to $\frac{1}{2}$ cup morning and night on the second day, if necessary. This tea usually takes 8 hours to work.

Note: If you have high blood pressure, omit the licorice root. Talk to your health care provider before taking any laxatives if you are pregnant or breast-feeding. This tea is for those 10 years and older. Never take a laxative if you're having severe abdominal pain.

Chapter 6

Helping and Healing
the Skin

T he skin is our body's largest organ and serves as the
interface between our internal and external world. It
gives rise to our sense of touch, the only sense that
does not diminish with age. Because our skin is what
we present to the world, billions of dollars are spent every year
on creams, lotions, and cosmetic surgeries. I have long been fascinated with the world of skin care, learning a great deal about
the physiology of the skin from the researchers and product
developers at companies such as Bath and Body Works, Neu-
trogena, and Origins, with whom I've worked as a consultant
over the past 20 years. In exchange, I shared my knowledge of
how plants could be used to restore barrier function and reduce
oxidative damage, inflammation, and irritation. But over the
many years I've cared for those with skin problems, I've also
learned that it takes more than just applying moisturizer to
have healthy skin.

Before we dive into the herbs and remedies, it might be useful to spend a few minutes talking about the basic anatomy
and function of the skin. The skin is made up of three parts:
the outer layer, known as the epidermis; the middle layer, or

dermis; and an underlying layer of subcutaneous fat. The epidermis is where vitamin D is absorbed and initially synthesized and where the pigment melanin—which gives our skin its color and protects it from the damaging effects of the sun's ultraviolet rays—is produced.

The cells in the epidermis are tightly packed to prevent the entry of bacteria and to preserve the moisture-holding properties of the skin. As cells travel from the base to the top, lipids are secreted to "fill in" the gaps between our cells. These lipids are made of fatty acids, cholesterol, and ceramides, which are vital for maintaining the barrier of the skin. Without adequate lipids, cracks develop between the cells, allowing bacteria to gain a foothold, thus triggering a local immune and inflammatory response. The abnormal production of these lipids is one characteristic of atopic dermatitis (AD), or eczema, and why essential fatty acids, such as evening primrose oil, can benefit people with AD by improving barrier function.

The thick layer of tissue found beneath the epidermis is what one might consider the "true" skin because it is where the blood vessels, nerve endings, sweat glands, hair follicles, and other structures are found. The nerve endings in the skin are highly sensitive to pain, pressure, and temperature. For instance, when we are cold, a coordinated effort between the muscles, blood vessels, and nerves causes the tiny muscles at the base of our skin hair to contract, making the hair stand erect, forming goose bumps. Air is trapped between the erect hairs and the skin, creating insulation and warmth. When we are hot, we sweat to cool off. Without this ability to regulate our body's temperature in hot weather, we would perish from heatstroke.

There is always a risk for infection if our skin is cut or damaged. The body defends against this via the secretion of antimicrobial proteins (AMP) by cells in our skin and sweat glands. These AMP are capable of killing many bacteria, viruses, and fungi, and are also important for triggering an immune response if harmful organisms should penetrate the skin. These proteins are essential for both preventing and clearing infections. Although good hygiene is important, our modern obsession with showering, hand-washing, and antiperspirants may not be such a good idea. Excessive washing decreases the barrier function of our skin and washes away these important AMP, increasing the risk for inflammation, irritation, and infection.

The nerves in our skin are also highly sensitive to our emotions. Our ancestors observed this for centuries, giving rise to expressions such as "he really gets under my skin." Have you ever noticed how your skin seems to glow when you're on vacation and how dull it can look when you're feeling overwhelmed? Well, scientists have shown that stress causes the release of chemicals that alter the barrier function of our skin. This loss of barrier function causes the skin to feel drier, wrinkle more easily, and trigger flares of eczema in vulnerable individuals. I cannot remember a single patient with psoriasis or atopic dermatitis who didn't believe that stress made their condition worse. Knowing this relationship, however, opens the doorway for improving the health of your skin by developing strategies to better manage stress. (See Chapter 4 on the nervous system.)

● Skin Microbiome

You may not realize it but your skin is actually a highly complex ecosystem that provides a home for trillions of bacteria, viruses, and fungi. Researchers at the National Institutes of Allergy and Infectious Diseases have shown that these microbes are absolutely essential for the skin's defense systems. One friendly inhabitant— *Staphylococcus epidermidis,* for example—acts to stimulate the production of AMP, which helps keep down populations of harmful microbes.

Although we live harmoniously with many microbes on our skin, they can sometimes cause trouble. Take, for example, the bacteria *Staphylococcus aureus* ("staph"), found on the skin of up to 30 percent of healthy people. If the skin is damaged, even with a minor cut, these bacteria can cause infection. Sometimes these infections can be quite serious because so many staph strains are now resistant to the antibiotics penicillin and methicillin, hence the term methicillin-resistant *Staphylococcus aureus* (MRSA). It may shock you to know that, according to the Centers for Disease Control (CDC), more people in the United States now die of MRSA than of AIDS. This is why having healthy skin is important, and why good wound care is critical if the skin's barrier should be breached. You want to prevent small problems from becoming big problems.

Herbalists have been dealing with wounds since ancient times. Many plants are rich in antimicrobial compounds that destroy *S. aureus, E. coli,* and a whole host of other pathogens that can cause skin infection. Of the 300 medicinal herbs that German health authorities have evaluated, 47 were for dermatological conditions! And as you will see in reading this chapter, herbs can be used to reduce inflammation, ease itching, and promote healing.

◗ The Rise of Allergic Skin Disease

Eczema is a general term used to describe many types of skin inflammation (dermatitis). Atopic dermatitis (AD) is the more specific name for a chronic type of eczema that is often accompanied by asthma or allergies. It's shocking that up to 20 percent of young children in western Europe and the United States have AD. That's three times more than 40 years ago. We've also had an almost identical rise in asthma and allergies. These three conditions are linked and are collectively referred to as atopic disorders, or atopy. Atopy is a type of allergy in which the hypersensitivity reaction can occur in a part of the body that is not in contact with an allergen. For example, individuals with atopic disorders who are allergic to dairy may experience an outbreak of eczema behind their knees or have an asthma attack. Individuals who do not have atopic reactions would have a localized effect in their gastrointestinal tract (for example, diarrhea or stomach cramping).

What is causing this dramatic increase in AD? Well, as I alluded to in Chapter 2, many researchers believe that life is much "cleaner" than it used to be. The numbers and types of microbes we come into contact with have dramatically changed. Many of our modern practices, such as drinking pasteurized milk, eating irradiated food, giving children more than 24 vaccines before the age of five, the indiscriminate use of antibiotics in people and livestock, and even the way babies are born and fed, have dramatically changed our microbial environment. Far more AD is present in modern, urban society than in rural society. (Note: I AM in favor of childhood immunizations, as I believe their benefits far outweigh their risks.)

In what is known as the hygiene hypothesis, it is thought that without early exposure to "the dirty side of life," our immune system is not properly trained to distinguish harmless from harmful. Without the ability to discern the difference, our immune system begins to see innocuous substances, like cat dander, pollen, or even our own cells, as something dangerous.

For good health, it is important that our skin function optimally. Trouble spots, such as rashes or eczema, can develop, and wounds and insect bites can breach the integrity of skin. The good news is that you can take many natural approaches to deal with these problems. In this section, we'll start with managing atopic dermatitis, skin rashes, fungal infections, and acne. And then I'll teach you how to manage wounds at home, as well as to prevent and treat bug bites.

▶ Eczema: Consider Natural Alternatives

Over the years, I've treated many children with atopic dermatitis (AD) or what most people call eczema. AD is a skin irritation that causes dryness, itching, and redness. In more severe cases, the irritation will become so bad that the skin weeps and crusts, increasing the risk for infection and scarring. Eruptions usually occur in the bends of the joints, cheeks, and chest, although they can pop up anywhere. Of those with AD, 85 percent develop symptoms in their first year of life, and 95 percent will have symptoms by the age of five. It's really rare for someone to develop AD for the first time after age 30.

In Western medicine, AD is primarily viewed as an overactive immune response. Therefore, treatment focuses mainly on suppressing the immune system. This is why physicians prescribe topical steroid (cortisone) and anti-inflammatory creams, as well as oral antihistamines and steroids. The stronger the immune suppression, the more effective the drug is at relieving the rash. Although these medications improve the rash, the AD often returns when you stop taking them, and chronic use of topical steroids can thin the skin and reduce barrier function. More importantly, though, these medications are primarily dealing with what you see on the surface when the problem is happening at a much deeper level.

AD is a condition of nature and nurture, meaning that it has both genetic and lifestyle components. If one parent has eczema, hay fever, or asthma, the child has a 50 percent chance of also having one of these conditions. But dietary, lifestyle, and emotional factors are at play, as well.

Studies show that roughly one-third of children with AD are allergic to cow's milk products. Other common food allergies include eggs, soy, wheat, and tree nuts. You can take all the medicine in the world to suppress the skin reaction but if you're allergic to a food, you cannot fix the problem until you remove the offending agent. A holistic approach is the only one that makes sense.

Is It a Food Allergy?

The best way to identify food allergies is to do an elimination diet, in which all suspicious foods are completely removed from the diet for two to three weeks and then reintroduced one at a time for three days to see if symptoms reappear. Once, I cared for a three-year-old child with recurrent ear infections and AD who'd already had five rounds of antibiotics and frequently used topical cortisone creams to get the rash under control.

We took the child off all dairy products for two weeks. Then I had his mother reintroduce dairy products by having him drink a cup of milk three times a day for three days. Nothing happened the first 48 hours, but on the third day, he developed a stuffy nose, his ear started to hurt, and his skin erupted. After keeping him off all dairy products for one year, he was like a different child. The ear infections, skin flare-ups, and dark circles under his eyes were gone.

Food allergy testing can be done, but studies show that the elimination diet is still the "gold standard" for identifying problem foods. Find a dietitian or health care provider who is skilled at designing an elimination diet to help you, especially for a child under the age of two.

Restore Digestive Health

I've seen big changes in the skin when we focus on enhancing digestion and restoring the microbiota in the gut. For children with AD who are three years and older, I commonly use a children's bitter for a minimum of six to eight weeks. I put one five-year-old girl on these bitters, as well as probiotics and a topical herbal cream, after she'd been treated repeatedly with antibiotics and cortisone creams to control her eczema. After about eight weeks, her skin was clearing and the itch and irritation were gone. Even after witnessing this multiple times, I am still amazed at how closely digestion and the skin are connected.

I carefully selected each of the herbs in the children's bitter formula for their specific benefits. Dandelion gently enhances all aspects of digestion, so that dietary fats, starches, and proteins are more completely digested, reducing inflammation and restoring the healthier barrier function of the small intestine. Both dandelion and burdock contain the prebiotic inulin, which feeds the healthy microbes in the gut. Oregon grape root reduces small intestine bacterial overgrowth, a potential problem in

Children's Bitter Glycerite

10 grams dandelion root
10 grams chamomile flowers
10 grams burdock root
5 grams Oregon grape root
5 grams fennel seed
225 milliliters vegetable glycerin
95 milliliters water

Grind the herbs to a coarse powder and put in a saucepan. Add glycerin and water. Cook on the lowest heat setting, covered, for 20 minutes. Remove from heat and let steep for 10 minutes. Pour into a glass container. Cover with a lid. Shake well. If there is not enough liquid, add another 30 milliliters glycerin and 10 milliliters water. Let sit and shake daily for 2 weeks. Then strain, bottle, and label.

How to Use:
3 to 5 years of age: 15 drops before meals (up to 3 times a day)
6 to 8 years of age: 25 drops before meals (up to 3 times a day)
9 to 12 years of age: 50 drops before meals (up to 3 times a day)
12 to 15 years of age: 1 to 2 teaspoons before meals (up to 3 times a day)
15 years and older: 1 tablespoon before meals (up to 3 times a day)

children who've taken antibiotics. Fennel aids digestion and prevents any intestinal cramping that may be caused by the bitters, while chamomile gently calms and soothes the nerves.

Probiotics

A growing body of research suggests that taking a probiotic can be beneficial for AD. One study of 38 people with moderate to severe AD found that taking *Lactobacillus salivarius* orally improved their symptoms and decreased the number of staph bacteria on their skin. This would reduce the risk for staph infection, which often happens because people, particularly children, scratch the itchy inflamed areas, leading to cuts and scrapes in the skin where staph can multiply.

Mothers can reduce the risk of their child developing AD by taking the probiotic *Lactobacillus* GG during the last month of pregnancy, as well as giving it to the baby for the first six months of life. I would strongly recommend this if either the mother or father has asthma, eczema, or significant food or seasonal allergies (one of the atopic disorders). A study of 474 infants followed for four years found almost a 50 percent reduction in risk of AD when moms and babies took probiotics as described previously. (See Chapter 5, pages 157–161, for more information on probiotics.)

Heal and Protect Your Skin

Whenever we get a cut or scrape, our main concern is infection because the skin's protective barrier has been compromised. But those with AD have even more risk than the rest of us. That's because they already have altered barrier function and their skin is heavily colonized with *Staphylococcus aureus,* which produces a protein, a superantigen, that acts as a potent activator of the immune system. High numbers of these bacteria on the skin increase the severity of AD by exacerbating skin inflammation.

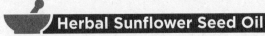

Herbal Sunflower Seed Oil

1 ounce calendula flowers
1 ounce St. John's wort, flowering tops
1 ounce chamomile flowers
18 ounces sunflower seed oil, organic

Grind the herbs into a coarse powder and put them in a glass jar. Add sunflower seed oil. Take a long-handled spoon and make sure that the oil moves freely in the jar. If it is too thick, add 3 to 6 ounces more oil. Repeat this process. Screw on the lid, put in a paper bag, and set in a warm, sunny place. If the oil is not completely covering the herb at any point, add more oil. Shake every day for 2 to 4 weeks. Strain.

How to Use: Apply this oil to affected areas every morning, night, and after bathing. Sunflower seed oil is excellent for maintaining barrier function.

Hygiene is important but don't overdo skin washing. Use glycerin soaps when bathing, because regular soap can deplete the natural lipids in the skin. Hot water robs skin of its oils, so take short, warm showers or tepid baths. Moisturizers are vitally important for enhancing the barrier function of the skin and should be used three to four times a day.

Both this Herbal Sunflower Seed Oil and my Natural Anti-Inflammatory Cream (recipe, pages 293–294) contain highly effective ingredients for enhancing the barrier function of the skin, reducing inflammation, and decreasing the colonization of bacteria. Although I love almond and macadamia nut oils, I generally avoid using them, or other nut-derived oils in those with AD, as more than a few are sensitive to them.

Sunflower seed oil has anti-inflammatory effects and restores barrier function by enhancing the natural lipid production of the skin. One study found sunflower seed oil was far superior to a petroleum-based ointment for preventing infections in premature babies in newborn intensive care. It is highly moisturizing and helps maintain the protective barrier function of the skin.

German chamomile has been used in a proprietary cream for eczema in Germany since the 1920s. Studies have shown its anti-inflammatory effects to be similar to over-the-counter cortisone cream but without adverse effects. The German health authorities approve of the topical use of chamomile for treating inflammatory conditions of the skin.

St. John's wort and calendula have antibacterial activity, reducing bacterial colonization and acting as potent anti-inflammatories. A double-blind study of 21 people with AD found St. John's wort cream to be highly effective at relieving inflammation and itch. This Herbal Sunflower Seed Oil can be used just as is, or it can form the base for the Natural Anti-Inflammatory Cream.

Natural Anti-Inflammatory Cream

I prefer to use creams, not salves, oils, or ointments, for red, blistering areas. Creams are a little harder to make, so you may want to purchase an herbal cream made from licorice, calendula, chamomile, and/or other soothing herbs from the local health food store or natural grocer. If you're up for a little adventure, though, you can make this one at home. (See the recipe in Chapter 9, "The Eighteen Essentials," pages 293–294.)

The little five-year-old girl I mentioned earlier in this chapter used this cream every day for a few months and then a few times a week, or as needed, for years thereafter. Unlike steroid creams that can cause thinning of the skin with persistent use, this cream has no adverse effects. It's absolutely amazing for relieving itch, soothing irritated skin, and increasing the skin's natural barrier function.

Coconut Oil

Coconut oil has long been used to moisturize the skin. I'm a fan; that's why I use it in my Natural Anti-Inflammatory Cream. It's an excellent moisturizer and has powerful antibacterial properties. One study showed that staphylococcal colonization *decreased by 95 percent* in people with AD when they applied coconut oil to their skin twice a day for four weeks!

How to Use: Take a small amount of organic virgin coconut oil and rub into affected areas twice daily.

Evening Primrose Oil

Evening primrose is high in the essential fatty acid gamma-linolenic acid (GLA). More than 30 studies have shown that evening primrose oil (EPO) is highly beneficial for AD. A study of 1,207 patients found that orally consumed EPO helped relieve itching, crusting, and redness. This is likely because it helps restore lipid balance in the skin, reducing local inflammation. EPO has been studied in both children and adults.

How to Use: The dose is 2 to 8 grams a day of evening primrose oil standardized to contain 8 to 10 percent GLA. Increase the dose based upon age and severity of the condition. I find little benefit until you get up to doses of 3 to 4 grams a day in children and 6 to 8 grams a day in adults.

Note: If you are taking prescription blood thinners, do not take more than 2 grams a day of EPO without first talking to your health care provider.

➕ Seek Medical Attention Now for Eczema

- If skin becomes swollen or painful
- If skin shows signs of yellow drainage or pus
- If skin has red streaks extending out from affected area

◐ Red Bumps and Itchy Spots: Skin Rash Treatments

A rash is technically an area of reddening, sometimes with raised spots, that appears on the skin. It can be localized or widespread, and it can itch, burn, swell, tingle, blister, or not be associated with any discomfort at all.

The causes of rashes vary. They can be triggered by a virus, like shingles; a fungus, like ringworm; or bacteria, such as impetigo. You can develop a rash from an insect bite, or a parasite like scabies. Sometimes a rash is caused by cold, dry weather, or at the other end of the temperature spectrum, heat rash. On very rare occasions, a persistent rash that won't go away may indicate a more serious disease. Because there are just too many rashes to put in a short chapter, I'm going to focus on just a few, though the treatments recommended will work for most.

Irritant Dermatitis

Dermatitis, which literally means "skin inflammation," occurs either from direct irritation by an external substance or an allergic reaction to it. (We discussed atopic dermatitis, an allergic reaction not caused by direct contact, on pages 204–205.) If the rash is around your hairline, you may be sensitive or allergic to something in your hair dye or shampoo. A more generalized rash may be due to sensitivity to a new fabric softener or detergent. A rash around your wrist could be an allergic reaction to the nickel in your new bracelet. After a day in the woods, that rash on your leg might be an allergic reaction to poison ivy. In general, allergic reactions are usually delayed and itchy, whereas irritant dermatitis is more immediate (your skin turns red and inflamed on contact) and hurts more than itches. When possible, try to identify the offending agent so you can avoid it in the future.

If you think you have been exposed to an irritant, I suggest using a vinegar wash to remove as much of the irritant as possible.

Apple cider vinegar is a versatile, neutralizing agent. Some recommend using it undiluted, but I've found it can be irritating to skin that is already red and inflamed. You can also just use plain soap and water if you don't have apple cider vinegar. The point is this: You want to dilute any irritant that might be on your skin!

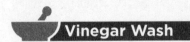

Vinegar Wash

1 cup apple cider vinegar
2 cups water

Mix both ingredients together. Rinse the area with the vinegar wash to remove as much of the irritant as possible. Let your skin dry.

||||||||||||||||||||||||||||||||||||||||||||||||||||||||||||||||||||||||||||||||||||||||||||||||

☎ Call Your Health Care Provider
- If your rash worsens in 24 to 48 hours, despite basic treatment
- If a rash is painful
- If you have any skin blemish/mole that has become irregular, darker, or is changing in appearance

||||||||||||||||||||||||||||||||||||||||||||||||||||||||||||||||||||||||||||||||||||||||||||||||

Red, Itchy Rash

If a rash is itchy, red, or blistering, after rinsing with vinegar or water, you will want to apply a neutralizing poultice, which can be made from ingredients right in your kitchen cabinet. Oatmeal has been used for centuries as both porridge and medicine, particularly for skin problems. Oats contain many active ingredients, including a group of compounds called avenanthramides, that block the release of inflammatory compounds and histamines,

R℞ PRESCRIPTION FROM DR. LOW DOG
Grindelia for Poison Ivy
and Poison Oak

Grindelia was widely used by Native Americans for relieving the pain of poison ivy and poison oak dermatitis and was included in pharmaceutical medications in the early 1900s. I know of nothing more effective for this type of contact dermatitis than grindelia tincture (recipe, pages 283–284). You can apply it directly to a rash or mix it in with a small amount of calendula ointment or in an oatmeal poultice. Grindelia rapidly relieves itching and redness. If you live in an area where these plants are bountiful, keeping some grindelia tincture on hand makes good sense.

dramatically reducing redness and itch. Oatmeal has antiviral and antifungal activity, as well, making it useful for relieving the itch and pain of chicken pox, shingles, and ringworm. I add a small amount of baking soda or cornstarch to augment the skin-soothing and itch-relieving properties of oatmeal. See the recipe for Oatmeal Relief in "The Eighteen Essentials," pages 292–293.

Diaper Rash

It's no wonder babies get diaper rash, considering the prolonged exposure of their sensitive skin to moisture and irritants found in stool and urine. Diaper rashes can be mild or quite severe. The best way to prevent a diaper rash is to keep your baby's bottom dry. Change diapers frequently. Use unscented wipes or plain water to clean the area. If using disposable diapers, experiment to find the one that fits best—poor-fitting diapers cause irritation and give bacteria a foothold. If you are using cloth diapers, add ½ cup apple cider vinegar to the rinse cycle and avoid using strong detergents.

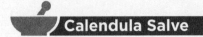
Calendula Salve

1 cup dried calendula (pot marigold) flowers
2½ cups sunflower seed oil
4 ounces grated beeswax

Put herbs and oil in a Crock-Pot on its lowest setting and cook for 8 hours. Turn off heat and let cool. Strain through cheesecloth. Pour 2 cups of strained oil into double boiler and add grated beeswax. Gently melt, stirring frequently. Dip a spoon into the mixture, lay the spoonful on a paper towel, and stick it in your refrigerator for 5 minutes. Take it out and test the consistency. If it's mushy, add 1 to 2 tablespoons more grated beeswax. If it's too hard, add 2 to 3 tablespoons more of your infused oil. (This is why we always make a little extra.) Test again. Texture should be firm. Pour into small glass containers or salve tins. Let completely cool and harden before putting on the lid.

Treating Diaper Rash

Wash your baby's bottom gently with water and blot dry. If your baby's bottom is looking bad, put ½ cup Oatmeal Relief in a small tub and fill with tepid, not hot, water. Let your baby play for 15 to 20 minutes in the tub. Then blot dry and apply calendula salve. A study found calendula salve highly effective for healing diaper rash. Calendula not only helps to heal the tissue, but it also reduces the risk of yeast and bacterial infection. Plus, the salve acts as a natural barrier against moisture. After applying the salve, place your baby on a towel with bottom up to expose it to air for 30 to 45 minutes. This entire process should be repeated twice a day. I also recommend giving the baby the probiotic *Lactobacillus rhamnosus* GG. It can be easily added to breast milk or formula.

Heat Rash

Heat rash looks like tiny pink or red dots or pimples and is caused when sweat ducts become blocked and swell. This rash is common in infants, because parents often bundle their babies up in the middle of summer. To prevent heat rash, don't overdress your baby. Adults can also get a heat rash in hot, muggy climates. The rash usually clears up within a couple of days without doing anything. The Oatmeal Relief bath can help soothe your skin if itchy.

✚ Seek Medical Attention Now for Skin Rash

- Some medications can occasionally cause a severe allergic reaction known as Stevens-Johnson syndrome, with a rash that often blisters. Ulcers start in the mouth and can form in the respiratory tract. You should SEEK IMMEDIATE MEDICAL ATTENTION if you are taking a medication and develop a rash with mouth ulcers.
- A child with a high fever, lethargy, and a rapidly spreading rash that turns into purple bruising should be TAKEN IMMEDIATELY to the emergency room, as this might indicate a *meningococcus* infection.
- If any rash is accompanied by shortness of breath or difficulty breathing
- If red streaks extend outward from the affected area
- If any rash is accompanied by a fever of 103°F or higher
- If a baby less than two months of age develops any rash, other than a diaper rash
- If a rash develops and spreads after being bit by a flea or tick

▶ A Fungus Among Us: Jock Itch, Ringworm, and Athlete's Foot

When I was eight years old, a couple of round, itchy rings appeared on my legs. My mom knew instantly what it was—ringworm—and then spent ten minutes reassuring me that I didn't actually have worms in my leg. People did once believe that it was caused by worms, hence the name. Ringworm, also known as *tinea*, is caused by dermatophytes, fungi that infect skin, hair, and nails. These fungi feed on keratin, a protein in the skin, and they only infect the outer layer of the skin. Jock itch, athlete's foot, and ringworm are all tinea infections.

Fungi grow and thrive in hot, moist areas. This explains why they often occur in the groin area, armpits, between the toes, or under a woman's breasts. Highly contagious, these infections are spread by sharing towels, combs, or brushes; walking around in public showers/locker rooms; or handling infected dogs or cats.

To prevent jock itch, athlete's foot, or fungal infections under the breasts, make sure you wash the area with soap and water and then dry thoroughly. Do NOT share towels. Wear loose-fitting clothing and natural fibers.

Neem Oil

I'm a huge fan of neem *(Azadirachta indica),* an evergreen tree that grows in the more arid regions of India, Southeast Asia, and parts of Africa. The seeds are used to make oil rich in potent antifungal and anti-inflammatory compounds. Research shows that it can effectively destroy 14 different types of dermatophytes, making it an amazing remedy for *tinea* infections.

Neem oil is commercially available in this country. Over the years, I have recommended it to many patients who have reported fantastic results for fungal infections, as well as scabies. The main drawback to neem is that it does not smell good. OK, it smells bad. Some companies have worked to improve the odor, but this is an issue you'll have to sort out for yourself. Neem soap is a great idea if you're prone to jock itch or athlete's foot.

Tea Tree Oil

Tea tree *(Melaleuca alternifolia)* is a small tree native to the northeast coast of New South Wales, Australia. Indigenous peoples of Australia used the leaves for treatment of fever, wounds, and as a beverage tea. The leaves are also used to produce tea tree oil. The first written medical testimony to tea tree was published in the *Medical Journal of Australia* in 1930, describing how the oil was used in surgical wounds. The oil was issued to soldiers during WWII as a disinfectant. Today, research has demonstrated that tea tree oil has considerable antifungal and antibacterial activity. One study found that both 25 percent and 50 percent tea tree oil solutions were highly effective for the treatment of athlete's foot when applied twice a day. I've used and recommended a blend of tea tree oil and witch hazel tincture for years.

||||||||||||||||||||||||||||||||||||||||||||||||||||||||||||||||||||||||||||||||||||||||||||||||||||||||||||||||||||||||||||||

☎ Call Your Health Care Provider

- If your rash worsens or does not respond to home remedies

||||||||||||||||||||||||||||||||||||||||||||||||||||||||||||||||||||||||||||||||||||||||||||||||||||||||||||||||||||||||||||||

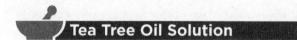

Tea Tree Oil Solution

2 tablespoons (30 milliliters) tea tree oil
3 tablespoons (45 milliliters) witch hazel tincture
3 tablespoons (45 milliliters) water

Pour the witch hazel tincture into a dark bottle and add the tea tree oil. Cover with a lid and shake well. Label the bottle "EXTERNAL USE ONLY."

How to Use: Apply to affected area 2 times a day. This recipe is a 25 percent solution. You can increase the tea tree oil to 90 milliliters for a 50 percent solution; however, this can be irritating for sensitive skin.

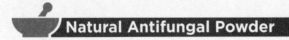

Natural Antifungal Powder

½ cup baking soda or cornstarch
4 drops tea tree oil
4 drops thyme essential oil
4 drops oregano essential oil

Put the ingredients in a jar and shake well to mix the oils and baking soda. Make your powder in small batches to preserve the power of the essential oils. Optional: If you live in a hot, humid area, add ½ teaspoon rice kernels to the powder to prevent clumping.

How to Use: Shake some of the powder into socks and shoes daily. You can also apply this powder under your breasts or to the groin area, especially after showering, if prone to yeast.

▶ Managing Acne: Lifestyle and Cleansing Choices

Acne is one of the most common skin conditions that drive people to the dermatologist. The reason some people experience acne is because of hormonal imbalances that lead to the overproduction of sebum, a lubricating oily substance that plugs hair follicles in the skin, creating a microenvironment that allows for the overgrowth of bacteria. Plugged pores (blackheads and whiteheads), pimples, and deeper lumps (cysts or nodules) can occur on the face, neck, chest, back, shoulders, and upper arms. These are acne-prone areas because they contain a high number of sebaceous glands, the glands that secrete sebum into the hair follicles and lubricate the skin and hair.

Anyone who has gotten beyond adolescence knows that hormones can have a dramatic impact on our skin's health and appearance. The skin becomes oilier after puberty, as androgenic hormones rev up sebum production, allowing a foothold for the acne-causing bacteria, *Propionibacterium acnes,* to proliferate. Women who are prone to acne often see a flare seven to ten days before their period. This is, in part, because progesterone rises mid-cycle, increasing sebum production and water retention, making the skin puffy and pores more compressed.

Acne generally starts between the ages of 10 and 13 and lasts for up to ten years, normally disappearing during the early 20s, though it can last longer in some. Ask anyone who has struggled with acne and you'll find that it can be emotionally traumatizing, harming self-esteem and confidence, particularly during the turbulent teenage years. And in a somewhat self-perpetuating cycle, high emotional stress aggravates the skin's barrier function, making it even more irritated and inflamed.

A number of acne treatments are available. Topical benzoyl peroxide is often used for mild forms of acne and, although effective, it can cause dryness and irritate sensitive skin. For more moderate acne, oral antibiotics are prescribed—usually tetracycline or doxycycline—taken between 3 and 12 months. Side effects associated with antibiotic use include bacterial resistance, alteration in the gut microbiome, and vaginal yeast infections. Many dermatologists prescribe isotretinoin (Accutane) for the treatment of severe, cystic acne. Again, although highly effective, isotretinoin can cause severe birth defects if a woman should get pregnant while taking the drug, so birth control is absolutely essential. Other side effects include skin and mucosal dryness, cracking or peeling of the skin, hair loss, depression, severe diarrhea, liver damage, joint pain, and more.

Treatments for acne must be individualized, but using the least harmful remedies first just makes common sense.

The Role of Diet

Just about everyone believes that eating certain foods can make acne get better or worse. The best evidence to date suggests that high-glycemic-load diets, meaning lots of refined carbs and dairy products, aggravate acne. A diet high in refined carbs can lead to insulin resistance and increased androgenic hormones, which explains why teenagers who drink soda and eat French fries, candy bars, doughnuts, and potato chips may fare worse.

Populations that eat healthy meats, veggies, and fruits with few refined carbs and dairy have a very low incidence of acne. Three studies in the *American Journal of Clinical Dermatology* have reported a link between milk and acne. One study found that teens drinking more than two glasses of milk each day had a 44 percent greater chance of developing severe acne. This may be due to the hormones present naturally in cow's milk that mimic androgen-like hormones in our body. And cows that have been given bovine growth hormone to increase milk production secrete a powerful growth hormone called insulin-like growth factor-1 (IGF-1) into their milk. IGF-1 has been shown to increase the production of sebum.

Although there are links between dairy and acne, there has been no association with *fermented* dairy. A 12-week study of 56 people with acne found that consumption of a *Lactobacillus*-fermented dairy beverage led to a significant reduction in total number of acne spots and a marked reduction in sebum production. It is hypothesized that the fermented dairy products improve skin health by normalizing the gut microbiome. Time and time again, I have found that when you improve the health of the gut, almost everything else improves to a greater or lesser degree. Think about adding a cup of probiotic-rich Greek-style yogurt or kefir, a fermented dairy drink rich in multiple *Lactobacillus* strains, to your daily diet.

There are numerous cookbooks and guides for how to follow a low-glycemic-load diet. In my previous book, *Life Is Your Best Medicine,* I wrote at length about this topic. This is by far the healthiest diet for many reasons, and the one I would recommend to those struggling with acne.

Cleansing the Skin

I cared for a 15-year-old boy who was really struggling emotionally with his facial acne. He had gotten into the habit of scrubbing his face with a washcloth, trying to strip away the bacteria and oil, leaving his skin even more reddened and inflamed. It's important to cleanse the skin but it must be done gently and not too frequently. I recommend using plain glycerin soap and water to wash the face once each day.

I've also been prescribing this Vinegar Green Tea Toner for more than a dozen years and have had fabulous results. Vinegar contains roughly 10 percent acetic acid, which gently exfoliates the skin, removes dead skin cells, dissolves the oil clogging your pores, and makes it hard for bacteria to thrive. Green tea has been shown to improve acne by decreasing sebum production.

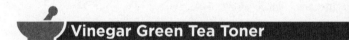 **Vinegar Green Tea Toner**

2 tablespoons (1 ounce) organic apple cider vinegar
3/4 cup (6 ounces) brewed green tea
1 teaspoon (5 milliliters) tea tree essential oil

Pour 6 ounces of near-boiling water over about 2 tablespoons (roughly three tea bags) green tea leaves and steep for 20 minutes. Remove tea bags. Pour into in an 8-ounce bottle, blend in other ingredients, shake well, cap tightly, and store in refrigerator. Use within a week.

How to Use: I suggest putting it on a very small area of the neck to make sure you don't have any sensitivity to the toner. If it burns or causes redness, wash it off immediately. If no problems, after washing your skin, pat dry and use a cotton pad to gently apply the toner. Allow it to dry and then apply your moisturizer. I recommend using it daily for 14 days for the most dramatic effects. Then you can use it 3 to 4 times a week, or as needed.

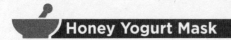

Honey Yogurt Mask

6 tablespoons probiotic-rich full-fat yogurt
6 tablespoons raw organic honey

Mix together and store in an airtight container in the refrigerator. Make sure to note the expiration date on your yogurt.

How to Use: Remove approximately 2 tablespoons from the container and set out on the counter for 15 to 20 minutes to warm up while you wash your face. Apply with your fingers or a clean cotton pad. Leave on for 10 minutes. Then rinse and apply moisturizer. Repeat 2 to 3 times a week.

Applying probiotics topically has shown to improve the skin microbiome and reduce acne blemishes. The raw honey is a potent antibacterial agent that can kill bacteria, while also moisturizing and nourishing the skin.

Tea tree oil has both antimicrobial and anti-inflammatory activity, making it a prime natural product to be studied as a topical agent for acne. One study of 124 people found that 5 percent tea tree oil gel was equivalent to 5 percent benzoyl peroxide lotion in ameliorating acne. The onset of action for tea tree oil was slower but it was better tolerated.

Digestive Health

Acne is the result of hormonal imbalances that are particularly common during the teenage years. Although it's not feasible to try to "lower" hormones, we can support the liver, which is responsible for deactivating and eliminating hormones. My go-to herbs in this case are dandelion root, gentian, and Oregon grape root. I recommend taking the Herbal Bitter Aperitif (recipe, pages 284–285) for 8 to 12 weeks before deciding whether or not it is helping. This formula also contains chamomile, which is soothing to the nerves, reducing anxiety and tension.

If you choose not to eat yogurt or drink kefir, I strongly encourage you to take a probiotic supplement that contains a variety of *Lactobacillus* species. And if you are taking antibiotics for your acne, it is imperative that you take a daily probiotic blend to keep those gut microbes in check. (See the introduction to Chapter 5 on GI health, pages 157–161.)

Blue Light

Patients have long reported that when their skin is exposed to the sun, their acne improves. Science has proven them correct. This is how it works: The bacterium that causes acne, *P. acnes,* produces porphyrins, substances that help bacteria to multiply in the skin. But the blue light of the sun causes the porphyrins to kill the bacteria instead. Ten minutes a day in the sun can be highly beneficial for those with acne, but if you are very fair skinned or concerned about the damaging effects of UV light, you can now purchase blue light devices without UV for home use. The evidence was strong enough that the FDA has approved the use of blue light therapy for the treatment of acne.

▶ Creepy Creatures: Treating Bites That Bug Us

My grandma Jo was severely allergic to bees. Whenever we'd get ready to go camping or fishing, my grandpa would ask, "Jo, you got the adrenaline?" as we climbed into his pickup. (We call that medicine "epinephrine" today, and it comes in easy-to-use self-administered injectors.)

Grandpa was right to be concerned. Death from bee stings is almost four times more common than death from snakebites, something I remind people when they visit our ranch in northern New Mexico. Insects inject venom made of protein and other compounds that not only cause pain and swelling but can also trigger an allergic reaction in certain people, like my grandmother. Severe allergic reactions, known medically as anaphylaxis, are thankfully relatively rare, but can cause hives, increased heart rate, weakness, and—most dangerous—can cause the throat to swell, making it difficult to breathe.

Stings from bees, wasps, hornets, and yellow jackets are most likely to cause allergic reactions, but other bugs can pose significant health problems. Ticks can carry Lyme disease and Rocky Mountain spotted fever. Mosquitoes can inflict the West Nile virus, malaria, dengue fever, and other diseases. Fleas can harbor bubonic plague. Lice can spread endemic relapsing fever, and deerflies can transmit tularemia. This is why it is important to protect yourself when going out in the woods camping, to keep indoor pets free of fleas and ticks, and to use mosquito repellent or protection if you live in an area where skeeters are a big problem. And if you are allergic to bees, make sure you always keep epinephrine on hand.

But before you go running indoors, I want to stress that insect bites are extremely common, and the vast majority of reactions are very mild. In general, the venom can make you itch, and you might get some mild redness and swelling, all of which improve in a day or two.

Bees, Wasps, and Fire Ants

Bees generally don't sting unless you infringe on their hive. More often, you step on one or get stung as you swat them. Honeybees lose their stinger along with their venom sac when they sting, so they can only sting you once.

Not so with bumblebees, wasps, hornets, and yellow jackets, however. For one thing, they're more likely to sting than

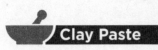
Clay Paste

2 tablespoons bentonite or French green clay
5 drops lavender essential oil
$\frac{1}{2}$ teaspoon arnica tincture
3 tablespoons water

Mix the arnica tincture, lavender essential oil, and water. Add slowly to the clay to make a paste. The clay helps draw out the venom from the sting and gets rid of the itch. The lavender essential oil and arnica dramatically relieve the swelling and pain.

How to Use: Apply the paste to the affected area. Cover it with plastic wrap or gauze for 30 minutes. Repeat this in 4 to 6 hours if needed.

I have used this Clay Paste so many times; it is amazingly fast and powerful for reducing pain and swelling from stings and bites.

---

honeybees. For another, they can keep right on stinging because they never lose their stinger! These stinging insects can be very aggressive if you're near their nest. Yellow jackets hang out around food and trash, so be extra watchful in those places.

Fire ants, or red ants, can pack quite an "ouch." Some people are allergic to fire ants, just like bees. The venom can cause significant swelling and pain, often forming a white pustule. Don't scratch it! That's how these bites become infected. Fire ants can bite repeatedly, and for such a tiny insect, their bites hurt.

Treating Insect Stings

1. If stung by a bee, remove the stinger if lodged in your skin. You can use tweezers, but the edge of a credit card works quite well, too.
2. Wash the affected area with soap and water.

3. Put a *cold* compress on the sting or bite as soon as possible. Remove it every 15 to 20 minutes. Leave off for 10 minutes and then reapply as needed. If you have witch hazel tincture on hand, put 2 tablespoons in 2 cups water and add ice. Swirl to make cold and use this instead of plain water.
4. Prepare a Clay Paste and apply several times a day, if needed.
5. Consider taking diphenhydramine (Benadryl, for example) to reduce swelling.

Spider Bites

In the contiguous United States, there are two poisonous spiders whose bites can be very serious: the black widow and the brown recluse. The black widow injects a toxin that poisons the nervous system. You may not even notice you've been bitten, but within a few hours, you'll feel stiffness and intense pain and swelling at the puncture site, and may develop fever, chills, nausea, and vomiting. You may need antivenin, which is available in most hospital emergency rooms.

The brown recluse, common in our desert Southwest, as well as in the Midwest, has a bite that produces a mild sting, local redness, and intense pain within six to eight hours. A fluid-filled blister forms at the puncture site, which sloughs off, leaving a

---

R︮X PRESCRIPTION FROM DR. LOW DOG

Scorpion Stings

Most scorpions in the United States are pretty harmless; however, the bark scorpion that lives in the desert Southwest can be dangerous if it stings a child or elder. If stung, wash with soap and water, put on a cold compress, and call your local poison control for advice, or head on over to the urgent care or emergency room. An antivenin called Anascorp is available, if necessary.

---

deep ulcer. Fever is relatively common, sometimes accompanied by nausea and vomiting. Although rare, children can die from the bite. As a physician in New Mexico, I've taken care of a number of brown recluse bites. The bites can be quite nasty. If either of these spiders is indigenous to your region, *learn to identify them so you know what they look like.*

If you think you have been bit by a black widow or brown recluse:
1. Clean the wound with soap and water.
2. Tie a snug (but not tight) bandage between the bite and your heart if the bite is on the arm or leg.
3. Apply ice to the bite and head to the hospital.

Treating Nonpoisonous Spider Bites

Now that I've filled you with fear and trepidation, I want to reassure you that the vast majority of the 50,000 species of spiders roaming the Earth don't cause significant harm to humans. The fangs of many are too small to penetrate human skin. Those that do inject venom through their fangs generally leave a small puncture wound that becomes red, itchy, and swollen.
1. Wash the bite area with soap and water.
2. Put a cold compress on the sting or bite as soon as possible. Remove every 15 to 20 minutes. Leave it off for 5 to 10 minutes and then reapply as needed. If you have witch hazel tincture on hand, put 2 tablespoons in 2 cups water and add ice. Swirl to make cold, and use this instead of plain water.
3. Apply Clay Paste as described previously.
4. Monitor for any signs of worsening pain, fever, or abdominal pain.

I was bitten by a brown recluse spider while out camping in southern New Mexico. We'd packed in and were about a two-day hike from our vehicles. I crushed some plantain, a great wilderness first aid plant, and applied it as a poultice, leaving it on for a couple hours. Because I had some echinacea in my pack, I dug up some red clay, added a little water to make it moist, and about a teaspoon of echinacea. I applied this makeshift clay poultice twice over the next two days, alternating with plantain. I am happy to report that the bite healed very nicely.

Mosquitoes, Deerflies, and Horseflies

Mosquitoes are by far the most common insect bite. You can do many practical things to help prevent bites, such as wearing light-colored long sleeves and pants, making sure your windows and doors have good screens on them, and draping mosquito netting over your child's stroller. But honestly, mosquitoes zero in on the carbon dioxide you exhale and are strongly attracted to certain scents, so unless you're going to give up breathing (which I don't advise) or using soap, there's no way to completely avoid these little critters.

Deerflies and horseflies are often a problem at my ranch. They can definitely make life miserable for the horses, and for us, when there's work to be done. They're mostly active during the day and are attracted to warmth, carbon dioxide, and movement. Their bites can be very painful. Sensitive folks may have an allergic reaction to the salivary secretions the insects release when they feed.

If I were heading out into the wilds of a dense tropical rain forest with swarms of skeeters or the woods with swarms of deerflies, no question, I'd be reaching for the DEET, short for N, N-diethyl-m-toluamide. DEET is highly effective for repelling mosquitoes but you want to follow the directions very carefully. If too much is absorbed, it can interfere with the central nervous system, causing impairment in motor and memory function. And more is absorbed than you might imagine, up to 17 percent of what you apply directly to skin. This is why children should not use any product containing more than 10 percent DEET applied only once a day. If using, spray it on your clothes, not skin, when possible.

However, for areas with more modest insect populations, I encourage you to make your own Natural Insect Repellent. A woman in Florida wrote me to say that she had difficulty with most mosquito sprays because they triggered her migraines. She said that my natural repellent worked great for keeping mosquitoes at bay and didn't cause a headache.

Treating Insect Bites

Mosquito bites are itchy and annoying but generally not serious. I was once bitten more than 100 times by mosquitoes in just one night on a camping trip in northern Michigan. I was miserable but fine. On the other hand, deerfly and horsefly bites typically cause more pain and swelling than mosquito bites. To treat these bites:

1. Wash the affected area with soap and water.
2. Put a cold compress on the sting or bite as soon as possible. Remove every 15 to 20 minutes. Leave it off for 5 to 10 minutes and then reapply as needed. If you have witch hazel tincture on hand, put 2 tablespoons in 2 cups water and add ice. Swirl to make cold, and use this instead of plain water.
3. Apply Oatmeal Relief to the affected area or use in your bath (see recipe, pages 292–293).
4. For a bad fly bite, use Clay Paste (recipe, page 227).

Tick Bites

Several close friends in New England have developed Lyme disease, and so I have heard about it firsthand, even though I don't live in a tick-infested area. Lyme disease is the most common tick-borne illness in North America and Europe. Roughly 25,000 cases of Lyme disease are reported each year in the United States. It is caused by the bacterium *Borrelia burgdorferi,* which is spread by infected deer ticks. If the infection is left untreated, it spreads through the bloodstream and lymph nodes, infecting the joints, nervous system, and possibly even the heart. One of my friends received antibiotic treatment within two weeks of the tick bite and was better quickly. My other friend thought he had the flu and so didn't receive antibiotics until almost two months after the tick bite. His joint pain lingered for months.

Although not as common, the most serious tick-borne illness in the United States is Rocky Mountain spotted fever (RMSF), which is spread by wood and dog ticks infected with the bacteria *Rickettsia ricketsii*. Although these bacteria were first discovered in the northern Rockies, RMSF occurs in many areas of the United States. Symptoms typically include a high fever and a "spotted" rash, which starts out as small, flat, pink, nonitchy spots on your wrists, forearms, and ankles that turn pale when pressure is applied. Over time, these spots become raised, and the skin eventually begins to turn black,

Natural Insect Repellent

1 cup (8 ounces) almond or sunflower seed oil
¼ teaspoon lemon eucalyptus
⅛ teaspoon geranium essential oil
⅛ teaspoon lavender essential oil

Put the almond oil in a bottle, add the essential oils, and shake well.

How to Use: Apply a small amount of the oil on your arm and leave for 30 minutes to make sure you are not sensitive to any of the ingredients. If no reaction occurs, then apply to exposed skin every 3 to 4 hours when you're outdoors. Avoid contact with the eyes, mouth, and nose, and do not use on children under the age of three.

hence its original name, "black measles." If untreated, RMSF can be fatal.

So what are these tick creatures anyway? Well, they are technically arachnids, relatives of spiders that live in woody areas. They survive by eating blood from animals or people. Ticks are most active in the United States from April through September, and it's important to be vigilant when hiking, camping, or playing in wooded areas and fields in areas where ticks are endemic.

For camping or hiking, I recommend wearing clothing that has been pretreated with either pyrethrin or permethrin, both of which are lethal to essentially all insects. Pyrethrin is a natural product derived from chrysanthemums, and permethrin is a synthetic, man-made form of this compound. These insecticides are widely used by the military when deploying soldiers into areas where mosquito-borne illness is high. They are also extremely effective for killing ticks and fleas. Only small amounts are needed to kill an insect, far less than what would be harmful to humans. In clothing, there is very little absorption into the skin or loss in water. Many manufacturers have tested their clothing and shown them to be effective for up to 70 washings. You could also spray a 20 percent DEET product for adults or 10 percent for children onto your clothes and exposed skin.

It's really important to shower soon after coming indoors, and look for any ticks that might have come home with you. Make sure to look in the bends of knees, arms, in the belly button, around the ears and especially in the hair. Parents should carefully look over young children. Throw your clothes in a dryer on high heat to kill any ticks. And if you took Fido with you, make sure you look him over carefully, too.

If you've had a tick bite, make sure you watch for any of the symptoms listed at the end of this section (page 234). The earlier you are treated with antibiotics, the better your chance of a complete and full recovery.

Removing a Tick

If you find a tick attached to your skin, don't panic. Use tweezers to grasp the tick as close to the skin's surface as possible and then pull up with steady, even pressure. Do not twist, or the mouth may be left in the skin. If this happens, remove it with the tweezers. After you remove the tick, wash the bite area with soap and water, or better yet, an Herbal or Essential Oil Wash, page 238. Don't try to remove the tick by using alcohol, a lit match, tobacco, or petroleum jelly. Either flush the tick down the toilet or save in a closed container for identification.

|||||||||||||||||||||||||||||||||||||||||||||||||||||||||||||||||||||||||||||||||||||||||||||||||||||||||||||||||

☎ Call Your Health Care Provider

- If you develop a rash, fever, fatigue, chills, muscle or joint aches, and/or swollen lymph nodes within several weeks of removing a tick, you should PROMPTLY see your health care provider. Another hallmark of Lyme disease, common but not universal, is the development of a rash around the tick bite that looks like a bull's-eye, with a red outer ring and clear center.

- If you live in or are traveling in the western part of the United States, where bubonic plague is found, and suspect a flea-bite, make sure you promptly see your doctor if you develop fever, chills, headache, and/or swollen lymph nodes.

|||||||||||||||||||||||||||||||||||||||||||||||||||||||||||||||||||||||||||||||||||||||||||||||||||||||||||||||||

Fleas

When I was a medical student, I spent four months working with Alan Firestone, M.D., at El Pueblo Health Services in Bernalillo, New Mexico. One day, he asked me to come into the examination room to see a patient. He pulled back the cloth drape, showed me a swelling in the groin area, and asked me if I knew what it was. I recognized that it was a swollen lymph gland but didn't know what had caused it. He then calmly told me it was a "bubo." Because I was still puzzled, he guided me outside the examination room and told me the patient had bubonic plague. I remember just standing there. The plague? What? We sent the patient to the University of New Mexico for antibiotics and treatment, and I was promptly instructed to learn all about the transmission and progression of bubonic plague.

Some of the most deadly plagues the world has ever seen were caused by the transmission of the bacteria *Yersinia pestis,* from fleas that had fed on infected animals, usually rodents, and then had bitten humans. Cats that eat an infected rodent can also transmit the plague through infectious droplets of saliva or other fluids. Someone infected with bubonic plague develops the sudden onset of fever, chills, headache, weakness, and one or more swollen, tender, and painful lymph nodes (called buboes). The bacteria multiply in the lymph node closest to where the bacteria entered the human body. While very serious, antibiotics can effectively treat the plague.

Fleas are small, wingless, armored, dark reddish brown insects that have powerful hind legs enabling them to jump several feet.

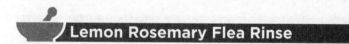

Lemon Rosemary Flea Rinse

1 lemon, sliced
10 drops rosemary essential oil
16 ounces hot water

Pour near-boiling water over sliced lemon (with peel and seeds) and steep, covered, overnight. Strain. Add rosemary essential oil.

How to Use: After shampooing and rinsing your pet, use a towel to remove most of the water and then take a sponge and apply the Lemon Rosemary Flea Rinse to the pet's hair and skin, especially around the tail, underarms, and around ears and neck. Allow your pet to dry naturally. It works really well.

There are many species of fleas in the United States, and they can be really difficult to eradicate once they gain a foothold in a house. If you find your dog or cat scratching, carefully look through their fur, especially at the base of the tail. You may not see a flea, but if you find small, black particles on the skin, that's flea feces.

Many people are rightfully concerned about the powerful flea products made from organophosphates and carbamates, chemicals that can cause seizures, nausea, and vomiting in your pet. Some natural flea products are available in the marketplace, most based on either pyrethrin from chrysanthemums or d-Limonene, from citrus. I would strongly encourage you to talk to your vet about what is safest for your companion.

In addition to treating your pet, however, you will need to thoroughly clean your home from top to bottom. Vacuum every nook and cranny, and make sure you remove the vacuum cleaner bag and put it in a tightly closed plastic bag after each use! Wash your pet's bedding in hot water and/or put in the dryer for 30 minutes—the heat will kill the fleas.

✚ Seek Medical Attention Now After a Bite or Sting

Call 911 or seek emergency medical assistance if you have any of the following signs or symptoms after a bite or sting:

- Difficulty breathing
- Swelling of the lips or throat
- Faintness
- Dizziness
- Confusion
- Rapid heartbeat
- Hives
- Nausea, cramps, and/or vomiting
- Fever
- Severe pain

Bathe your dogs with a good shampoo and then use the Lemon Rosemary Flea Rinse to kill off any fleas that didn't drown. Be careful here—do not use excessive amounts of essential oils on your pet! Follow this recipe carefully.

▶ More Than a Bandage: Sure Cures for Wound Care

Life is filled with cuts, scrapes, and bumps. I live on a ranch, so I am constantly taking care of minor mishaps. I've treated all kinds of wounds, whether human or animal, and we've had some doozies.

I've also taken care of many wounds and bites when working at the urgent care and emergency room (ER). Many definitely needed evaluation and treatment. For instance, a wound that is "dirty" with pieces of glass or deeply embedded rocks or dirt or one in which the bleeding cannot be controlled with direct pressure are best treated by a health care professional. A deep puncture wound, such as from a nail, may require you to get a tetanus shot if you haven't had a booster in the last ten years. Any bite from an unknown animal should also be evaluated.

But I've also taken care of many wounds in the ER that could've easily been tended at home. I often felt bad because people would wait for hours to have a clinician wash a wound, apply some antiseptic ointment and a bandage, and send them out the door with a large co-pay or bill. That's not a good use of anyone's time or resources. To help you discern whether you should attempt to treat the wound at home or head to the local urgent care, I've included a list of things to watch for at the end of this section.

I want to reassure you that a healthy body is well designed for staving off infection and healing itself. One of the first things you notice when you hurt yourself is that the injured area feels warm and becomes red—a hallmark of inflammation. This is when inflammation is a good thing: It is a sign that the body

Herbal or Essential Oil Washes

Here are a number of washes you can use, depending upon what you have in the cupboard:

2 teaspoons (10 milliliters) tea tree OR rosemary OR lavender essential oil
1¼ cups (300 milliliters) bottled or clean water

OR

2 tablespoons (30 milliliters) goldenseal OR Oregon grape root OR sage OR echinacea tincture
1¼ cups (300 milliliters) clean water

OR

30 milliliters witch hazel tincture OR yarrow tincture (use if bleeding is an issue)
300 milliliters clean water

Mix the tincture or essential oil and water together. Pour into a squeeze bottle and irrigate the wound. Repeat until the mixture is gone.

---

is sending nutrients and immune cells to the injury, removing waste and bacteria, and stimulating wound repair.

When treating minor wounds at home, remember two primary goals: Prevent infection and promote healing. Here are the steps for each.

How to Prevent Infection

Step 1: Thoroughly clean the wound with water or an herbal wash. If the wound is dirty, it's important to flush out bacteria, dirt, and other debris. A large 60-milliliter syringe is the best tool for this; you can pick up one at any pharmacy. Otherwise, keep a good squeeze bottle in the kitchen. Wash the wound repeatedly with small bursts of water/herbal wash. This is THE most important part of wound care.

Step 2: Next, wash the skin all around the edge of the wound with soap and water. Let the skin dry for 5 minutes.

Step 3: Use the T's Wound Salve (recipe, page 240), raw honey, or sage honey (recipe in "The Eighteen Essentials," pages 291–292). Apply the salve or honey to a clean gauze dressing and tape it over the wound. You may want to keep some adhesive strips, sometimes called butterfly bandages (for example, the brand Steri-Strips), on hand for those cuts that don't need stitches but where you want to bring the edges together for better healing.

Honey to the Rescue

Move over aloe vera. Raw honey is one of the best treatments we have for wounds and burns. When applied topically, honey is able to pull out debris, infection, and bacteria from wounds while drawing in white blood (immune) cells. The white blood cells contribute to a faster healing process. Honey dressings keep wounds moist and prevent gauze from sticking. Honey is amazing for "road rash" types of injuries. Make sure you use raw, uncooked honey.

How to Use: Paste about ½ ounce honey on a 3 x 3 gauze pad and apply, making sure to completely cover the wound and the surrounding skin. I generally cover this with a 4 x 4 gauze pad and secure with first aid tape, or use a waterproof bandage to keep the honey from oozing through the underlying gauze pad. Change the dressing daily. You can also purchase MediHoney dressings that are premade and ready to use on wounds.

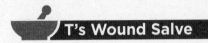

T's Wound Salve

10 grams goldenseal root or barberry root bark
10 grams calendula flowers
5 grams yarrow flowering tops
5 grams echinacea root
240 milliliters olive, grape seed, or sunflower seed oil (carrier oil)

Grind your herbs, put them into a glass jar, and add the carrier oil. Let it steep for 2 to 4 weeks. Strain, retain the oil, and compost the herbs.

We're doing a little variation on the salve, as I like to use raw honey in my wound salves.

2 ounces grated beeswax
4 ounces raw honey
50 drops tea tree oil
1 teaspoon vitamin E oil (optional)

Put the strained oil in a double boiler and slowly add grated beeswax, while gently stirring. Check and adjust for consistency. Remove from the heat. As it begins to harden, stir with an electric handheld blender until it is smooth. Let it cool for another 5 minutes, blending periodically. Now add your raw honey, vitamin E oil, and tea tree oil and continue mixing for an additional minute. Pour into salve containers and store in a dark, cool place.

How to Use: This salve is amazing for any kind of minor cut, scrape, burn, or for fungal infections such as athlete's foot. It is an all-purpose healing first aid salve.

This salve has been a mainstay in my practice and in my home for decades. Minor wounds heal faster and with less scarring.

How to Promote Healing

If a wound is minor, meaning not very large or deep, all you need to do is keep it clean. Change the bandage daily. This also allows you to watch for any signs of infection. Either pus or redness that seems to spread beyond the wound edges indicates a possible infection. Antibiotics may be required. I want to stress that this is not common if a wound has been properly irrigated and kept clean.

If there is swelling, you should keep the area elevated and apply ice to the affected area for the first 24 to 48 hours. Remember, ice for 10 to 15 minutes and then remove for 10 minutes to encourage healthy circulation and waste removal.

✚ Seek Medical Attention Now for a Cut or Wound

- If you cannot control the bleeding after ten minutes of *sustained, steady, firm* pressure. Most people stop pressure after only a few minutes, but most bleeding will stop if you don't let up the pressure for ten minutes!
- If you're unable to adequately clean the wound because of embedded glass, metal, or other debris
- If the injury resulted from a deep puncture wound, such as stepping on a nail
- If the wound appears deep or "gaping" and you think it's going to need stitches
- If you suspect a nerve or tendon was damaged; for instance, if you cannot move a finger or your skin feels numb
- If you suspect there is a broken bone
- If there was an animal or human bite
- If the wound appears infected; for example, it has a bad odor, redness, and/or pain that is increasing in intensity
- Consider going to the urgent care if you are taking medications that may suppress your immune system (for example, steroids or chemotherapy), if you have a disease/disorder that would make it hard for your wound to heal (for instance, diabetes or cancer), or are over the age of 75.

Chapter 7

Women's Medicine

As a midwife, physician, woman, and mother, caring for and connecting with women has always been near and dear to my heart. I've been privileged to journey alongside girls when they first enter the mystery of womanhood, attend women as they brought their children into the world, walk next to women as they moved beyond their childbearing years, and sit at the bedside of those as they journey to the other side. Through it all, I've learned that women carry a healer within them. Throughout history, from ancient times to the present, across cultures and ethnicities, we have always been the ones to tend the sick and broken, bring babies into the world and raise them, and provide comfort to the dying. It is women who keep our culture and families alive.

I believe most women are intuitively drawn to natural medicine. Surveys from countries around the world support this observation. Women repeatedly say that they want a greater say in their treatment, they would prefer to use gentle remedies first, and they want more personal control. I agree. Rare are the women who need to take prescription antidepressants to manage premenstrual syndrome. Although hormone therapy can alleviate menopausal symptoms, their use has been associated with an increased risk of blood clots and breast cancer. There are other options for women who have milder symptoms. A review by the international Cochrane Collaboration found that women who had midwives for their prenatal care and birth were significantly more likely to have a spontaneous vaginal birth, initiate breast-feeding, and feel in control.

Women have been the keepers of healing ways and the secrets of plant medicines. It is a part of our lineage. It is our birthright. I encourage you to learn as much as you can about how to care for yourself and your loved ones using gentle and effective means of treatment. We must educate ourselves about the risk factors for disease—which are primarily diet and lifestyle—and be proactive in taking steps to reduce our risk. We need to know when to reach out for the surgeon's hand and when things are better cared for at home.

I know that this can be hard. There's so much to do already. We often feel pulled in a thousand different directions. And one of the biggest challenges we face today is trying to figure out how to live a balanced life. I don't mean a life without ups and downs—but one that is resilient during change. We can start by going back to the basics. That means eating a wholesome diet and saying no to junk food, and making time to exercise, whether that means going to the gym or walking 30 minutes every day after lunch. We are spiritual beings and must nourish that part of ourselves, creating space for gratitude, joy, and reflection. Women often tell me they are too busy to exercise, too busy to cook, too busy to make time for themselves. They have too much to do. They have to take care of work, home, family.

I am a frequent flier on Southwest Airlines. Whenever we get ready to take off, the flight attendant comes on the microphone to provide us with safety information. "If we should happen to lose cabin pressure, oxygen masks will drop down from the panel above you. Make sure you put your own mask on first before assisting your child or someone else who might need help." Great analogy. You must make sure you are getting oxygen first, so that you will be conscious to help those around you. As women, we must take care of ourselves first. It's not selfish. It's absolutely necessary.

I've written an entire book on women's health and have edited another. It is beyond the scope of this book to dive deep into women's health, but I do want to share with you some of the things I've learned over more than 30 years of caring for women. In this section, we'll explore some of the more common problems women face, such as premenstrual syndrome (PMS), menstrual cramps, bladder infections, as well as some practical tips for having a healthy pregnancy.

▶ Monthly Woes: Mending Menstrual Cramps

I still remember my girlfriend Becky rolling up into a ball and crying on the first day of her monthly period. Her pain was palpable, and I felt so sorry for her. On top of that, our physical education teacher would never let her sit out class on those dreaded days. Only 12 at the time, I saw firsthand just how much a woman could hate her cycle. Becky wasn't alone, however. Menstrual cramps affect over 50 percent of menstruating women.

As a physician, I've learned how to help women prevent or dramatically reduce the impact of menstrual cramps, but it helps to understand what causes them in the first place. Menstrual cramps occur when there is an imbalance in chemicals called prostaglandins (PG) in the uterus. PGF2-alpha and PGE2 are pro-inflammatory prostaglandins involved in uterine contractions that occur during menstruation and labor. Without these PG, the uterus would not be able to contract and shed its lining during menstruation. These inflammatory PG are normally kept in check by PGE1 and PGE3, which act to inhibit uterine contractions. Women who produce excessive amounts of PGF2-alpha/PGE2 and/or not enough PGE1/PGE3 experience painful cramps.

Medications like ibuprofen, naproxen, and aspirin alleviate menstrual cramps because they block the production of pro-inflammatory prostaglandins. And although these medications are relatively safe when used on occasion, they do increase the risk for gastric bleeding. This is because they reduce blood flow to the stomach and duodenum, thinning the protective mucus layer that lines these organs, making them more vulnerable to the harmful effects of stomach acid. If using one of these analgesics for menstrual pain, chew 1 to 2 tablets of DGL (deglycyrrhizinated licorice, a special form of licorice) with each dose. DGL has been shown to help protect the stomach in those taking these types of analgesics.

These analgesics can temporarily relieve the pain, but they do not get at the underlying problem of excessive inflammation. You can do a number of things to shift your body's production from PGF2-alpha/PGE2 to PGE1/PGE3. Start by following a low-glycemic-load (GL) Mediterranean-style diet. The best way to eat a low-GL diet is to focus on getting your carbohydrates from fruits, vegetables, and whole grains. Skip the white bread, white potatoes, potato chips, white rice, spaghetti, soda, and processed foods.

Essential Fatty Acids

Fatty acids are acids produced when fats and oils break down. Essential fatty acids (EFAs) are those that must be obtained in the diet because the body cannot make them on its own. EFAs play an important role in regulating pain, inflammation, and swelling, as well as regulating smooth muscles (like the uterus), and much more. The most important EFAs are the omega-6 linoleic acid (LA) and the omega-3 alpha-linolenic acid (ALA). ALA is converted to eicosapentaenoic acid (EPA) and PG3. LA is converted to dihomo-gamma-linoleic acid (DGLA) and then can be converted to either PG1 or into arachidonic acid (AA), a precursor of PG2. If there is not enough omega 3 fatty acid in the body, LA is converted to AA.

The evidence shows that the American diet is woefully low in omega-3 fatty acids, which are found in fish, nuts, and seeds, such as flax, pumpkin, and walnut. The American diet is also very high in omega-6 fatty acids, found in vegetable oils like safflower, sunflower, corn, and soybean. These oils are found in large quantities in many processed and prepackaged foods. The ratio of omega-6 to omega-3 in the American diet is roughly 16:1. Ideally, it should be closer to 3–4:1.

Omega-3 fatty acids shift the production of prostaglandins from the pro-inflammatory to the less inflammatory. In other words, you will make less PGF2-alpha and more PGE1 over time. There are three primary omega-3 fatty acids: eicosapentaenoic acid (EPA), docosahexaenoic acid (DHA), and alpha-linolenic acid (ALA). Fish contains EPA and DHA. Nuts and seeds contain ALA, which must be converted to EPA and DHA, a process the human body does relatively inefficiently. This is why most researchers recommend either eating fish or taking fish oil supplements to lower inflammation.

Several studies have shown that taking 1 to 2 grams a day of fish oil for just three months can dramatically reduce menstrual cramping. For this reason, I strongly recommend that women with menstrual cramps take a fish oil product that provides 800 to 1,200 milligrams a day of EPA and 400 to 800 milligrams a day of DHA in the fewest number of pills. Store your fish oil capsules in the freezer and take with your largest meal of the day as dietary fat enhances absorption.

If you are a vegetarian and do not want to take fish oil, you can take flaxseed oil capsules that provide at least 2,000 milligrams a day of ALA.

Magnesium

Magnesium is wonderful for reducing menstrual cramps, as well as easing menstrual-related headaches and the flu-like feeling some women experience right before their period. Magnesium is a natural muscle relaxant and is necessary for the production of PGE1 in the body. Foods rich in magnesium include dark-green leafy vegetables, beans, nuts, seeds, and whole, unrefined grains.

Take 400 to 600 milligrams every day, not just during menstruation.

Note: If you have poor kidney function, do not take supplemental magnesium without first speaking with your health care provider.

Dong Quai: A Gift From Asia

Dong quai is a fragrant perennial found throughout China, with related species in Japan and Korea. The roots of this plant have been used in traditional Chinese medicine (TCM) for more than 20 centuries for a variety of ailments, including menstrual pain, scanty periods, and as a female tonic. The drug company Merck introduced the herb to the Western world in 1899, under the trade name Eumenol, a product that was said to positively affect menstrual disorders. Modern science confirms that dong quai exerts significant anti-inflammatory and analgesic activity, which would explain why it is one of my absolute favorite herbs for women who have light periods with painful cramps.

Note: Dong quai should not be used during pregnancy or if you have heavy menstrual bleeding.

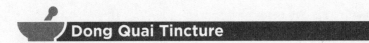

Dong Quai Tincture

25 grams dong quai root
125 milliliters brandy (80 to 100 proof)

Grind the herb and put the grounds in a jar. Add brandy. Put a lid on tightly. Let the mixture steep in a warm place for 2 to 4 weeks. Strain and put the liquid in a dark-colored jar, label, and store in a dark cabinet.

How to Use: Take 1/2 teaspoon of tincture every 4 to 6 hours, as needed for menstrual cramps.

Black Haw or Cramp Bark: A Gift From North America

Cramp bark and its cousin black haw have long been used by indigenous peoples of North America and early American physicians to prevent miscarriage and relieve painful menstrual cramps, leg cramps, after-birth pains, muscle spasms, and asthma. Both herbs were so widely used and recognized for these purposes that they were officially entered into the *United States Pharmacopoeia* in 1882, and remained in the *National Formulary* until 1960.

Over the years, I've used black haw and cramp bark to relieve menstrual cramps in hundreds of women. Both herbs work wonders, especially when taken in conjunction with daily magnesium. Cramp bark will often relieve leg cramps when all else fails. And I've seen a number of pregnant patients use it to prevent miscarriages.

These herbs are so effective that I've been disappointed that researchers haven't taken a greater interest in studying them. What science does show is that both herbs attach weakly to "beta-2 adrenergic receptors," which when bound, tell the uterine smooth muscle to relax, alleviating cramping. By the way, these same receptors are what cause the smooth muscles in the lungs to relax, supporting the historic use of this medicinal in the treatment of asthma as well.

While I was pregnant with my daughter, Kiara, I started having uterine contractions around my 16th week, quickly accompanied by a small amount of vaginal bleeding and some cervical changes that showed up on a physical exam. I was frightened that I might miscarry.

A few weeks earlier, a blood test had indicated that my baby might have Down syndrome. Well-intentioned friends told me it was "God's will" and "all for the best." My midwife encouraged me to rest and drink more fluids, which I did. I also started drinking ¼ cup of strong cramp bark tea four to five times a day. It worked like magic. The cramping would stop for five to six hours before gradually starting up again. I'd drink more tea and everything would quiet down, as if the tea had turned off a switch. Around

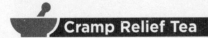

Cramp Relief Tea

1 tablespoon black haw or cramp bark
1$\frac{1}{2}$ cups (12 ounces) water

Put black haw or cramp bark in cool water and bring the mixture to a boil. Cover. Turn heat on low and simmer for 10 minutes. Turn off heat and let the mixture steep for another 10 minutes. Strain. Sweeten with honey, if desired. Store in your refrigerator for up to 3 days.

How to Use: Drink $\frac{1}{4}$ cup of tea every 2 to 3 hours, as needed, for menstrual cramps. For leg cramps, take $\frac{1}{4}$ to $\frac{1}{2}$ cup tea an hour before bedtime.

---

my 26th week, I was finally able to stop drinking the tea altogether. My beautiful Kiara was born at home, full-term and healthy.

▶ Let's Be Honest: Herbal Answers for Premenstrual Syndrome

Ever since I was a teenager, I've watched women struggle with the emotional and physical fluctuations that can accompany their periods. You know what I'm talking about: Your breasts become sore, your tummy feels like a beach ball that desperately needs deflating, and your sweet boyfriend or husband suddenly gets on your nerves for no reason. Technically, these monthly discomforts are called "premenstrual syndrome" (PMS). Most women experience PMS at some point in their lives, particularly when feeling under a lot of stress.

I once asked my Grandma Jo if she had ever had PMS. Puzzled, she asked me what it was. "You know, Grandma, when you feel kind of cranky and irritable a few days before your period starts," I said.

She gave me that old familiar grin, and with a twinkle in her eye said, "Oh sure, honey. I didn't know they had a name for that. I just thought those were the times I was being a little more honest with your Grandpa."

I've thought about that story many times as I've grown older. There was such simplicity in her answer. She didn't say she'd never felt that way, only that she had accepted it as a part of who she was. These days we are so quick to medicalize natural phases of womanhood such as menstruation or menopause. I believe there is a risk in always seeing every emotional or physical discomfort a woman experiences as something pathological. If we think we are sick, we shift our energy into a sickness mode, and this interferes with healing and well-being.

And, there are times when our "femaleness" can be used as a weapon against us. I was doing my internship at the University of New Mexico when one night, after being on call and awake for 37 hours, the attending surgeon decided he wanted to get something to eat before doing our evening rounds. That would have meant it would be at least another couple hours before we could go home. We were exhausted. I had an infant at home, and it just seemed ridiculous that we'd have to wait around for him. I asked if it would be OK if we rounded first so that our team could go home. He made some snide comment about maybe going out for a steak. I asked him why he had to be like that. He looked me right in the eye and said, "What's the matter, Low Dog? That time of the month?" I then said something I probably shouldn't have. But like my Grandma Jo, I was apparently suffering from an intense bout of honesty.

An Integrated Approach

Premenstrual syndrome is defined as a recurrent, cyclical set of physical and behavioral symptoms that occur 7 to 14 days before the menstrual cycle, and are troublesome enough to interfere with some aspects of a woman's life. Eighty percent of women experience some degree of premenstrual emotional or physical changes, but only 20 to 40 percent of these women report that it poses any real problem in their life.

The causes of PMS are not known. Hormonal, neuroendocrine, and nutritional factors are all likely at play. We know that stress can directly influence the production of hormones and neurotransmitters such as serotonin and dopamine. Women with PMS have been shown to have a decline in serotonin after ovulation, which may affect mood and sleep. Ovarian hormones influence calcium, magnesium, and vitamin D, and deficiencies in these nutrients can increase PMS. A deficiency of PGE1 in the central nervous system may also be involved, and transient elevation of the hormone prolactin can cause breast tenderness and moodiness.

One of the most promising areas of research involves the role of endorphins. Women normally have an increase in beta-endorphins, or natural opiates, in their bloodstream after ovulation. Women with PMS have lower levels of these circulating endogenous opiates. Symptoms such as anxiety, food cravings, headache, and physical discomfort are directly and inversely proportional to beta-endorphin levels in the body.

The reality is that PMS is multifactorial. I've found that lifestyle adjustments, herbal medicines, and natural supplements can have a balancing effect on the female system. Equipped with some simple remedies that have been used for centuries, you can easily turn things around so that your hormones no longer have the upper hand over your life.

Take Off the Edge

Stress dramatically worsens PMS, so make sure you are incorporating lifestyle strategies for keeping it in check. Regular exercise, yoga, a healthy diet, and getting enough sleep are good places to start.

Roller-coaster blood sugar can definitely worsen PMS symptoms. Prior to and during your period, shun sugary and processed foods that send your blood sugar soaring. They'll only end up making you feel tired, sad, and irritable—and craving even more junk food. Get off the white bread, white pasta, white rice, and sugary drinks and foods, and focus on eating lots of veggies, fruits, whole grains, and lean meats. Protein is crucial during this time. Cut your sweet craving with a protein smoothie in the morning, or some almonds in the afternoon.

Watch your caffeine intake, too. Studies have shown that caffeine can trigger anxiety and increase breast tenderness. If you drink four cups of coffee or cola a day, you'll need to cut back throughout the month, not just before your period! Sudden caffeine withdrawal can worsen irritability and trigger nasty headaches.

Don't forget the importance of omega-3 fatty acids, as was discussed at length in "Monthly Woes," pages 245–250. A deficiency in PGE1 may be involved in PMS, so make sure you include more cold-water fish like salmon, tuna, and halibut, and/or take a fish oil supplement that provides 800 to 1,200 milligrams a day of EPA and 400 to 800 milligrams a day of DHA. If you are a vegetarian, consider taking 2,000 milligrams a day of flaxseed oil.

Many herbs can help take off the edge. Chamomile, skullcap, and lemon balm are all wonderful for those few days before your period when you may be feeling more irritable or not sleeping as well. Many women find the Herbal Stress Relief tincture/glycerite to be an awesome ally during this time. (See the recipe in "Resiliency," page 131.)

Chasteberry: PMS Problem Solver

The dried fruits of the chaste tree *(Vitex agnus-castus)* have been shown repeatedly to relieve the symptoms of PMS and to normalize irregular menstrual cycles. Multiple studies have demonstrated that these berries reduce irritability, improve mood, and ease bloating and breast tenderness that often occur before the menstrual cycle. In fact, the German health authorities endorse chasteberry for PMS, breast tenderness/fullness, and menstrual irregularity. I absolutely adore this plant.

Chasteberry acts, in part, by reducing prolactin, increasing progesterone, and binding opiate receptors, preventing the decline in endorphins during the second half of the cycle. When elevated, prolactin can cause breast tenderness and even impair fertility, causing your periods to become erratic and making it difficult to get pregnant. And increasing progesterone stabilizes the uterine lining, regulating the menstrual cycle.

Chasteberry and Infertility?

Infertility is distressing and emotionally painful. But let me give you some comfort: Chasteberry may be helpful. Don't let its name fool you. Chasteberry, also known as monk's pepper, was used in very small amounts in food in the belief it would help monks maintain their vow of chastity. Ironically, though, the herb may actually enhance fertility. One reason is that it is involved in the process that increases progesterone. Higher progesterone may reduce the risk of early miscarriage.

During my medical training, one of the female residents asked if I knew anything that could help her get pregnant and stay pregnant. She'd been thoroughly evaluated in the wake of two prior miscarriages, both of which happened before her tenth week. Because no abnormalities were found, she and her husband were trying to conceive again. I recommended chasteberry, because I'd used it with good results in a dozen or so women over the years.

She took 2 milliliters chasteberry tincture (see the previous recipe) once each morning (about 400 milligrams of the dried fruits) for several months and became pregnant. She stopped taking it when she was 16 weeks pregnant. At the end of a full term, she had a beautiful, healthy baby girl. As to the scientific validity of

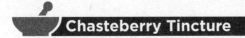

Chasteberry Tincture

25 grams chasteberries, dried
125 milliliters vodka (80 to 100 proof)

Gently grind the chasteberries in a clean coffee grinder and put them in a jar. Add the vodka. Put on lid, label the jar, and let it sit in a warm place for 2 weeks, shaking daily. Strain. Pour liquid into a clean bottle, label, and store in a cool, dark cupboard.

How to Use: Take 2 milliliters each morning for PMS or irregular menstruation. Chasteberry should be taken every day for at least 3 months to bring your hormones back into balance. I also recommend women take this for several months when going off birth control pills. The herb has an excellent safety profile, and women can take it safely for extended periods of time.

---

using chasteberry to overcome fertility, some research in Europe shows that chasteberry can be beneficial, but more research in this area needs to be done before it can be widely recommended.

Note: Work with a midwife or practitioner experienced in the use of herbs before relying upon them to become pregnant or during pregnancy. If you experience a sudden abnormal change in your menstrual bleeding, make an appointment to see your health care provider.

The Menstrual Minerals: Calcium and Magnesium

Some very solid science has shown that calcium can ease both the psychological and physical symptoms of PMS. In one study of over 400 women, for example, those who took 600 milligrams calcium carbonate twice daily reported an average 50 percent decrease in PMS symptoms over three months. Other studies have found similar benefits, which may reflect calcium's ability to ease the hormonal fluctuations that occur in the days before menstruation. I generally tell women to steer clear of calcium carbonate, as it is very constipating and may not be as easily absorbed.

Research has found that women with PMS have low levels of magnesium in their red blood cells compared to controls. Studies have shown that magnesium can ease PMS-related mood swings, as well as breast tenderness, water retention, and bloating. Magnesium is the treatment of choice to prevent migraines, particularly menstrual migraines. Magnesium is involved in muscle relaxation and in the regulation of serotonin, a neurotransmitter known to be involved in the onset of migraine headaches. Fluctuating serotonin levels in the brain can cause blood vessels to spasm, stretching delicate nerve endings and causing significant pain. This effect on serotonin explains why magnesium also benefits mood. If that's not enough, magnesium plays an important role in maintaining normal heart rhythm, blood pressure, and blood sugar levels. It also counteracts the constipating effects of calcium!

Look for a product that provides 300 milligrams of calcium citrate and/or malate and 300 milligrams of magnesium citrate and/or malate. A number of companies make these 1:1 blends. Take twice a day for a total of 600 milligrams calcium/

☎ Call Your Health Care Provider

- If you have emotional or physical premenstrual symptoms that interfere with your daily activities and life. If you feel markedly depressed or anxious before your period and self-care/home remedies don't make them better, make sure you talk to your health care provider.
- Before using ANY herbal remedy during pregnancy, talk to your midwife or doctor.

magnesium. I have found that women generally do not need to take 1,200 milligrams of calcium a day, the dose used in a number of the studies, if they eat a healthy diet and take the calcium with magnesium.

Note: Supplemental magnesium should not be used without medical supervision if you have poor kidney function.

◉ Flow-Through: Keeping Bladder Infections at Bay

I'm sure you'll never forget the last time you had a bladder infection, commonly referred to as a urinary tract infection (UTI). That stinging, agonizing, got-to-get-to-the-bathroom sensation is certainly no fun. If you've had a bladder infection, you're not alone. UTIs are the second most common type of infection in the body, right behind colds/upper respiratory infections. They are particularly common in women from adolescence through our elder years, as well as during pregnancy. In fact, up to 8 million women in the United States get a UTI every year. UTIs are relatively rare in men, but if a man gets one, it can often be serious. Because UTIs are so common, prevention is really important, and knowing how and when to use natural remedies for treatment makes good sense.

Since urine is normally sterile, you wouldn't think bladder infections would be so common. Here's what happens: An infection occurs when bacteria, usually *E. coli* from the intestinal tract, attach themselves to the opening of the urethra, the tube that drains urine from the bladder, and begin to multiply. If the infection stays localized in the urethra, it is called urethritis. Urethritis is often caused by *Chlamydia* and *Mycoplasma*, sexually transmitted organisms. If your infection is due to one of these organisms, you and your partner will both need to be treated with appropriate medication.

If the infection travels to the bladder, it is technically called cystitis. If not treated properly, the infection can spread to the kidneys, causing pyelonephritis, a far more serious condition. That's because from the kidneys, the bacteria can spread to the bloodstream, a condition called sepsis, which can be deadly. Roughly 40,000 people each year die from sepsis due to *E. coli*. Although most bladder infections are uncomplicated, they should not be taken lightly, particularly in young children, people over the age of 60, women who are pregnant, or someone with a compromised immune system, where the risk of kidney infection and sepsis is greater.

The best way to prevent UTIs is a healthy lifestyle. Drink plenty of water (six to eight cups of pure water daily) to keep the bladder flushed, and urinate when you feel the urge. And, if you're prone to bladder infections, take showers instead of baths. In addition to these basic "to-dos," the following strategies can be particularly helpful and may help you sidestep antibiotics.

℞ PRESCRIPTION FROM DR. LOW DOG
Know the Difference

Symptoms of a Bladder Infection (Cystitis)

- Sudden onset
- No fever, chills, or nausea
- No upper back pain
- Burning on urination, frequent need to urinate

Symptoms of a Kidney Infection (Pyelonephritis)

- Gradual onset
- Fever, chills, nausea
- Pain in upper back, on one side, upper rib cage
- Urinary symptoms (burning, frequency) may not be present

A Berry Good Cure: Cranberry and D-Mannose

Cranberry has been scientifically shown to reduce risk for getting a UTI. Cranberries, and probably blueberries, contain compounds that prevent bacteria from attaching to the lining of your urethra and bladder, making it hard for them to get a foothold or ascend up the urinary tract. Yes, you can drink cranberry juice as a preventive, but many people find it tedious to drink it every single day (not to mention that it's loaded with calories).

There is a better solution: cranberry extract capsules. A study comparing the cost and preference of women with recurrent bladder infections found that cranberry extract capsules were less expensive than juice and preferred by most.

Based on findings like this, I suggest purchasing a good brand of cranberry extract. Also, take it with D-mannose, a nondigestible sugar that acts as a decoy inside your bladder. *E. coli* attaches to the D-mannose rather than to the bladder wall and is flushed out when you urinate.

Take about 400 milligrams of cranberry extract with 500 to 1,000 milligrams of D-mannose twice a day. A number of excellent brands provide this level of both ingredients in two capsules. Cranberry and D-mannose are safe, even during pregnancy.

Barberry Barrier for Prophylaxis

Vaginal intercourse makes it easier for bacteria to reach the bladder through the urethra. The risk for bladder infection increases with frequent sex, which explains the slang expression "honeymooner's cystitis." For women in whom this frequently happens, physicians will often prescribe an antibiotic to be taken after sex for prevention. I'm generally reluctant to do this as it disrupts the body's microflora, increasing the risk for gastrointestinal problems, vaginal yeast infections, and growth of resistant strains of bacteria.

What I've found works for many women is to apply a tincture of barberry root bark or Oregon grape root bark around the urethra after intercourse (see the section on tinctures for the recipe). It's inexpensive, topical, and effective. For women who really struggle with recurrent bladder infections, I have them use this treatment as a preventive two to three times a week. Up on our ranch in northern New Mexico, we have hundreds of wild barberry plants *(Berberis fendleri)*. The roots are bright yellow, almost fluorescent due to the presence of berberine, an alkaloid found in other species of barberry *(Berberis vulgaris)*, Oregon grape root *(Mahonia aquifolium* or *Berberis aquifolium)*, as well as goldenseal *(Hydrastis canadensis)* and goldthread *(Coptis chinensis)*. Numerous studies have shown berberine to be highly active against *E. coli* strains, inhibiting their growth and blocking adhesion to the urethra and bladder wall.

How to Use: Apply the tincture with a clean cotton ball to the urethral opening (the opening where you urinate) after intercourse. Barberry can stain clothes and sheets, so it's usually a good idea to do this in the bathroom while seated on the toilet. The tincture dries quickly once applied. Use a clean cotton ball if you need to reapply.

Bladder Infection Protocol

Herbal therapies can be safely used to treat uncomplicated bladder infections in healthy, nonpregnant women. I have used the following protocol successfully in my practice for many years. It relies heavily upon the herb uva ursi, also known as bearberry, a highly effective antibacterial agent. Uva ursi *(Arctostaphylos uva ursi)* has been used as a diuretic and treatment for bladder infection and inflammation for centuries. The European Scientific Cooperative on Phytotherapy (ESCOP) lists it as "a treatment for uncomplicated cystitis where antibiotics are not warranted." Uva ursi contains the compound arbutin, which is broken down

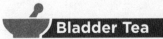

Bladder Tea

30 grams (about 1 ounce) uva ursi leaves
15 grams (about $\frac{1}{2}$ ounce) corn silk
4 cups (32 ounces) water

Pour 4 cups near-boiling water over the herbs and let the mixture steep for 20 minutes. Strain. You can store the tea for 2 days in a covered jar in the refrigerator.

How to Use: See pages 262–263 for recommended dosage.

If you live where you don't have easy access to purchasing herbs, you might want to get these herbs ahead of time and make them into a tincture to have on hand in case you need it. Tinctures will last many years.

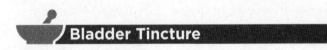

Bladder Tincture

25 grams uva ursi leaf
15 grams corn silk
200 milliliters vodka (80 to 100 proof)

Grind uva ursi and corn silk and put in a jar. Cover with the alcohol. If necessary, add another 40 milliliters vodka to ensure your spoon moves readily through the mixture. Let it sit, covered, and shake daily for 14 days. Strain. Pour into dark bottle, label, and store.

How to Use: See pages 262–263 for recommended dosage.

---

to hydroquinone in the urinary tract, where both compounds release their powerful antibiotic properties.

I also include corn silk, the long silky strands that you find when you peel the husk back from an ear of corn. Although it lacks the antimicrobial power of uva ursi, it soothes the irritation, pain, and burning that often accompany a bladder infection.

Here is the bladder protocol I have found to work:

The first 48 hours:

Drink ½ cup of bladder tea every 2 to 3 hours during the day (6 doses). The tea can be taken warm or cold. Sip slowly. OR if using tincture, take 3 milliliters in ¼ cup hot water or juice every 2 to 3 hours during the day (6 doses).

Mix 2 ounces of cranberry juice with 6 ounces of water and drink every 2 hours during the day (8 doses). Hydration is key to flushing out bacteria. Drink at LEAST this much fluid.

Take 200 milligrams of vitamin C every 2 to 3 hours during the day (6 doses). The extra vitamin C will help your body rid itself of the infection.

Most of the time, your symptoms will improve within 8 to 10 hours. If symptoms worsen or do not improve in 24 hours, you should see your health care provider. If symptoms improve, after 48 hours:

➕ Seek Medical Attention Now for Bladder Infection Symptoms

If you think you have a bladder infection AND:

- Are pregnant
- Are under the age of 12
- Are over the age of 65
- Are a male
- Have diabetes or kidney problems
- Have a weak immune system or take immune-suppressing drugs
- Have fever, chills, nausea or vomiting, or pain in one side of your back under your ribs

---

Days 3 through 5:

Drink ½ cup bladder tea 3 times a day OR take 3 milliliters bladder tincture in ¼ cup hot water or juice 3 times a day.

Mix 2 ounces of cranberry juice in 6 ounces of water and drink 4 times a day. You still need to stay hydrated. Drink plenty of water. Take 200 milligrams of vitamin C 3 times a day.

After 5 days, discontinue tea or tincture and continue drinking plenty of fluids and taking vitamin C for 2 to 3 more days.

Note: Uva ursi should not be taken longer than 4 weeks and should not be used by pregnant or breast-feeding women.

◖ A Special Time of Life: Natural Remedies for Moms-to-Be

As a physician, midwife, herbalist, and mother, I've experienced being pregnant and I've been privileged to walk beside and partner with women as they brought their children into the world. It is a special time in our lives, filled with a mixture of emotions—excitement about the life within us, and anxiety about what lies ahead. I've always believed that women have a special kind of courage to lie upon the birthing bed and bring life into the world. And I know that it takes even greater strength and courage to mother our children as they grow.

Whether a first or a fifth pregnancy, each journey is as unique as the child. Some of us will experience morning sickness, hemorrhoids, bladder infections, or insomnia, and then, of course, seasonal allergies, colds, stomach upsets, and other problems that may come along. It's important to consider the safety of whatever remedies you use while pregnant. Some prescription drugs, over-the-counter medications, and herbal remedies are not safe for your baby, especially during the first trimester. You should always talk with your midwife or doctor about any health concerns you have; however, I'd like to share with you some of the remedies

I've been recommending for almost 30 years. I trust their gentle and reliable therapeutic effects. So, in addition to your prenatal vitamin, you might want to consider some of the following.

Morning Sickness

I had morning sickness for only a few weeks when I was pregnant with my son. But wow, it was awful. I remember being able to find just one position one morning that didn't make me feel like throwing up. The slightest movement would bring on a wave of nausea so I just lay there for about two hours until it passed. Ugh. I tried to drink peppermint, but even the smell made me feel sick. Chamomile definitely helped but I sure wish I'd known about these next two options back then!

Vitamin B_6 and Doxylamine: The Dynamic Duo

A number of studies have shown that the combination of vitamin B_6 and doxylamine (an over-the-counter antihistamine) is highly effective for morning sickness. According to the American College of Obstetricians and Gynecologists, "taking vitamin B_6 or vitamin B_6 plus doxylamine is safe and effective and should be considered a first-line treatment" for relieving nausea and vomiting in pregnancy. It has been studied in more than 6,000 pregnant women with no evidence of harm to the babies. And more than that, some studies show that it improves the symptoms of morning sickness by 70 percent!

How to Use: Take 10 to 25 milligrams of vitamin B_6 every 8 hours. This is often enough just by itself. If you need more help, ask your pharmacist to help you find doxylamine in the store. The dose is 25 milligrams of doxylamine at bedtime, and 12.5 milligrams each in the morning and afternoon.

Tip: Sometimes, taking prenatal vitamins can worsen morning sickness. If so, I recommend switching to a children's chewable multivitamin. Just chew two at night before bed for a few weeks until you're feeling better.

Ginger

Ginger is a spicy culinary herb with a long history of relieving nausea and indigestion. When I was little, my mother and grandmothers would give us ginger ale to settle our stomachs. I guess they were on to something. Ten studies have shown that ginger is highly effective and safe for relieving moderate to severe morning sickness in pregnant women. And if that weren't enough, you can also reach for the ginger if you feel like you're getting a cold or want to relieve a stuffy nose while pregnant.

You can take ginger in a number of ways, but remember, dried ginger is a stronger antinausea remedy than fresh. It doesn't mean fresh won't work, just that the constituents responsible for settling your stomach concentrate upon drying. Fresh ginger, however, is awesome for colds!

Ginger candy: Some women love candied or crystallized gingers, which are yummy, effective, and easy to carry in a purse. Just eat or suck on one every few hours, as necessary, when that queasy feeling hits. I have used these on car trips when our daughter was young, as she would often get carsick. It worked like a charm!

Capsules: If taking capsules, make sure you purchase those that say they only contain ground ginger rhizome/root, usually 400 to 500 milligrams per capsule. You can take up to 1,000 milligrams of dried ginger a day. Many ginger products in the marketplace are highly concentrated ginger *extracts*. They are NOT safe in pregnancy.

Ginger tea: You can purchase ginger tea bags, which make preparation easy, especially when you already aren't feeling well.

Or you can make your own by pouring 1 cup of near-boiling water over ¼ teaspoon ginger powder. Let it steep for about 10 minutes and then pour off the liquid. Discard the powdered sediment. Sip on this tea, hot or cold, throughout the day. If you have a sore throat, you can use fresh or dried ginger. Add some lemon and/or honey, and you're good to go!

Ginger ale: Keeping a couple bottles of natural ginger ale in the cupboard is a good idea during the first trimester. Although I'm not an advocate of soda, I definitely make an exception in this case. The blend of ginger and carbonation is a winning combination for easing nausea. Just be aware that many commercial ginger ales only contain ginger flavoring, along with high-fructose corn syrup and other things you don't want. If you're going to use ginger ale for morning sickness, purchase "the good stuff" at a health food store or natural grocer.

Keep Your Bladder Healthy

Urinary tract infections (UTIs) are very common in pregnancy, which is one reason we check urine during prenatal visits. An untreated bladder infection can quickly turn into a bad kidney infection requiring hospitalization. An antibiotic is usually given if bacteria are detected in the urine, and if a second UTI occurs, prevailing practice is to put you on antibiotics for the rest of your pregnancy.

Make sure you drink plenty of water every day to stay hydrated. I suggest making spritzers with cranberry juice, which can help keep bad bacteria from attaching to the walls of the urethra and bladder. If you would prefer to take your cranberry in capsules, just look for one that will provide you with 400 to 600 micrograms of the extract, and take it morning and night. Remember, you want to try to *prevent* bladder infections. If you are pregnant, don't try to *treat* a bladder infection at home.

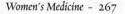

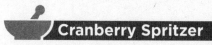

Cranberry Spritzer

2 cups cranberry juice (with no high-fructose corn syrup)
3 cups water, sparkling or still
1 orange, sliced

Mix the cranberry juice and water together and put in a pitcher.
Wash and slice an orange and add. Refrigerate.

How to Use: Delicious and refreshing, this drink can be served
cold over ice. Drink 1 cup twice a day.

Soothe the Burn

Heartburn is not uncommon, as the hormones of pregnancy
relax the sphincter at the top of the stomach, allowing acid to
creep back up into the esophagus. Practical tips include eating
smaller meals, eating slowly, and not eating before bed.

Calcium

Using chewable calcium (300 to 400 milligrams) to squelch the
burn not only works great, but the extra calcium is also good for
both you and the baby. But be careful not to overdo it. Taking
1 to 2 a day is plenty. Make sure you look for an antacid that
contains calcium. It's best to avoid those that contain aluminum
and nix the baking soda; it's notorious for causing swelling during pregnancy.

Slippery Elm

One herb that can be very helpful is slippery elm bark. It has
been used for centuries as a safe, delicious, and delightfully effective remedy for sore throat and heartburn, which is why I always
keep some lozenges on hand. Chew 1 to 2 tablets as needed.

Relax With Chamomile

German chamomile is one of the most gentle and beneficial plants I've ever worked with. The botanical genus name *Matricaria* is derived from the old French *matrice*, meaning "womb" or "uterus," hinting at its long and respected use during pregnancy. It quiets and calms, helping you relax after a long and chaotic day and making it easier to fall asleep naturally. It eases cramping and inflammation, making it a wonderful ally during pregnancy for occasional tummy upset, sore throats, and colds.

Chamomile tea: Make the tea according to the instructions under the section on teas and tisanes. Drink a cup in the evening to unwind, or drink ½ cup 2 to 3 times a day to settle an upset stomach.

Chamomile glycerite: Prepare this according to the instructions in the section on glycerites in "The Eighteen Essentials." Take 1 to 2 teaspoons in the evening to relax or several times a day to settle an upset stomach.

Note: There are no contraindications for German chamomile while pregnant or breast-feeding listed in the *German Commission E Monographs,* the *World Health Organization Monographs,* the *British Herbal Compendium,* or the *Botanical Safety Handbook.* Do NOT use Roman chamomile in pregnancy. One caution is the rare risk of allergy in those allergic to plants in the daisy family.

The Magic of Magnesium

Magnesium can ease those nasty leg cramps that sometimes happen in pregnancy, as well as help you to get a good night's sleep. Because magnesium has natural laxative properties, it can counteract the constipating effects of pregnancy and calcium supplements. It is also my number one choice for preventing migraines in pregnancy, when our pharmaceutical options are more limited (see the section on headaches). And last but not least, magnesium keeps our cells sensitive to insulin, making it particularly valuable for those who are at risk for gestational diabetes.

Take 400 milligrams about an hour before bed. Choose magnesium citrate or chelated magnesium for a mildly laxative effect, or magnesium glycinate if you have a tendency toward loose stools.

Vitamin D

Vitamin D is important for healthy bones for mom and baby, but you may not realize that if you're deficient in this important nutrient during pregnancy, it can increase the risk for pre-eclampsia, preterm labor, and gestational diabetes. It may also increase your baby's risk for developing type 1 diabetes and asthma. Your prenatal vitamin probably has 400 to 600 IU vitamin D_3 in it, though many experts, myself included, believe that the optimal dose is somewhere between 1,000 and 2,000 IU a day. Instead of guessing, however, it's best to ask your midwife or doctor to check your vitamin D level to make sure your level is somewhere around 30 nanograms/milliliter.

◗ Two Additional Supplements for the Last Trimester

When babies are inside the womb, their gastrointestinal tract is sterile. In the process of being born, the digestive tract is seeded with the bacteria present in the mother's birth canal. If the baby is breast-fed, scores of healthy bacteria are ingested through her milk. This is the foundation for good digestive health.

Probiotics

Probiotics are organisms that promote and maintain the natural balance of bacteria in the gut. A growing body of research shows that when mothers take probiotics during the last couple months of pregnancy, their children are given some protection against eczema, allergies, and possibly asthma. Babies born by C-section who are given probiotics after birth may gain some protection against these allergic tendencies.

But probiotics don't just benefit babies; they're good for mamas, too. A review of the best studies conducted to date shows that probiotics can help reduce the risk of gestational diabetes.

Yogurt: Look for yogurts that say "live and active culture," preferably those that contain *Lactobacillus acidophilus, L. casei,* and/or *L. reuteri.* Some yogurts are loaded with high-fructose corn syrup and sugars, so choose the healthiest you can find and eat one cup a day.

Probiotics: Look for products that contain multiple *Lactobacillus* strains such as *Lactobacillus acidophilus, L. casei,* and/ or *L. reuteri.* Either shelf-stable or refrigerated products can be used. Take as directed on the label for at least the last 12 weeks of pregnancy.

Fish Oil

Supplementing with fish oil during pregnancy has been shown to lower the risk of premature birth and increase the baby's growth and birth weight by improving blood flow across the placenta. It may also help reduce the risk for postpartum depression. Omega-3 fatty acids, particularly DHA, are highly concentrated in the baby's brain and eyes, and it's vitally important that sufficient amounts are on board during the last trimester of pregnancy, when neurological development is very rapid. Studies show that babies born to women consuming fish or fish oil during pregnancy score better on tests that assess intelligence, attention, and visual acuity than those born to women with little omega-3 intake.

Fish offers other health benefits as well. In the medical journal *Clinical Reviews in Allergy and Immunology,* researchers found that the majority of scientific studies show a reduction in the prevalence and severity of eczema, hay fever, and asthma in babies born to women who took fish oil during pregnancy.

Fish oil capsules: Take a high-quality fish oil supplement that provides 200 to 500 milligrams of DHA and 600 to 800 milligrams of EPA a day.

DHA-only supplements: If you are vegetarian or vegan, DHA supplements (the fatty acid so important to your baby) made from algae are available in the marketplace. Take 200 milligrams a day. Include ground flax or chia seeds, walnuts, and other foods high in omega-3 fats in your diet.

Raspberry: The Herb of Pregnancy

Hear the word "raspberry," and those delicious red berries picked in late summer or early fall come to mind. But there's more to the plant than the berry. The leaf of the red raspberry has been considered a "woman's herb" for centuries. Women have relied upon the tea to regulate menstrual cycles, ease menstrual cramping, and as a nutritive during pregnancy.

For many years, I drank raspberry leaf tea three to four times a week as a refreshing and tasty beverage. My periods were regular like clockwork, light, and pain-free. The trick with raspberry is to use it regularly over an extended period of time.

I also drank the tea during my pregnancies, and it appears I'm not alone. Surveys indicate that 15 to 25 percent of women in the United States, Canada, and Australia take raspberry leaf at some point during their pregnancy. A specific case in point: A survey of 172 certified nurse midwives found that 63 percent of midwives who reported using herbal preparations recommended red raspberry leaf to their patients. Raspberry leaf is listed as a Category A with the Therapeutic Goods Administration (TGA) of Australia (their version of our FDA) for use during pregnancy. This means that it has been used by large numbers of women without any increased harm to the baby.

A Natural Tonic: Nettle Leaf

You may know stinging nettle as an annoying plant with a painful bite. But did you know that it also has a prominent place in history?

The stalks of nettle were once widely used for making cloth to use for sheets, tablecloths, and clothing during World War I, when Germany and Austria ran low on cotton and turned once again to nettle to make cloth. And in Europe, young nettles were routinely enjoyed in the spring the same way many enjoy cooked spinach leaves.

Healthwise, nettle was widely used to ease arthritic pain and menstrual pain. Modern studies show that nettle has anti-inflammatory activity, which supports its historical use. Nettle leaves also dramatically reduce the activity of *E. coli* bacteria in the bladder, making it useful for minor urinary tract infections. And nettle leaf is a popular remedy for staving off seasonal allergies. A good source of calcium, iron, and other nutrients, it blends nicely in women's teas, particularly during pregnancy.

Like any leafy vegetable, nettle is extremely safe and nutritious. I grow it in its own little patch in my garden. When I'm ready to pick the leaves, I use gloves to prevent the hairy leaves and stems from irritating my skin. For a side dish, I steam them for 15 minutes and sauté in a little olive oil with garlic and salt. I also hang bunches of nettle leaf to use for medicine.

Nettle root is used to improve symptoms of enlarged prostate in men. Don't use it in pregnancy. I am ONLY speaking about nettle LEAF here.

Heart-Centered Tea

I am a firm believer in the power of healthy rituals in our lives. One that I have encouraged for many pregnant women over the years is the art of tea and journaling. I would mix these herbs, put them in a jar, tie a ribbon around the neck, and write in calligraphy her name followed by the words "Heart-Centered Tea." I would gift this to her and suggest that she get a journal and, starting at 34 weeks, drink a cup of tea and write letters to her child for 10 to 15 minutes every night. Lovely.

Women are highly sensitive and intuitive during the latter part of pregnancy. This is a wonderful way to channel that energy. I would like to encourage you to open up your heart in this way, too. Write about your life, your dreams, your fears, and your hopes for you and your child. Be vulnerable. On your child's 18th birthday, or whenever the moment is right, give him or her your heart journal. My son told me how it struck him that I was only a few years older than him when I wrote him those letters, that I seemed so young and yet so grown up. He hadn't thought of me in that way before. It was powerful for both of us. When I reread some of the letters, I realized that I could never have said

Heart-Centered Tea

2 cups raspberry leaf
1 cup nettle leaf
$\frac{1}{2}$ cup spearmint leaf

Mix all the herbs together in a jar with a tight-fitting lid. Label and store in a cool, dark cupboard.

How to Use: Pour 1 cup of near-boiling water over 1 to 2 teaspoons of the herbs and steep for 5 minutes. Strain. Add honey or lemon, if desired.

those things to him today, because I am a different person. A lot of life happened over those 18 years. And yet, I was filled with love for that young woman who carried that child and brought him into the world, who was brimming with love and hope, her youth shining from within. *You can never step into the same river twice.* Capture these precious moments now.

Shatavari for After the Birth

One of the gifts I always bring a new mother is shatavari, wild asparagus root, an herb from India that has been traditionally used to help women regain their strength after birth, help with the production of breast milk, and normalize hormones to protect against depression. Ancient Ayurvedic texts indicate that shatavari has been used medicinally for at least 4,000 years. Countless numbers of women have shared their love for this nourishing remedy.

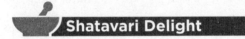

Shatavari Delight

60 grams shatavari root, dried
10 grams powdered cardamom
2 tablespoons raw sugar

Grind the shatavari to a coarse powder and then mix all the ingredients together and put in a jar with a tight-fitting lid. Label and store in a dark cupboard. This will keep up to 3 months.

How to Use: Put 1 teaspoon mix into a cup of milk, soy milk, or almond milk in a saucepan and gently bring to a boil. Turn off the heat, cover, and let steep for 5 minutes. Strain and drink once a day. Yum.

Chapter 8

The Gift of Plants

Human beings have been in relationship with the green world since the beginning of time. Our lives are dependent upon the plants. They recycle carbon dioxide and generate oxygen, providing the very air we breathe. Almost by magic it seems, they are able to convert sunlight into energy and then use soil and water to bring us a vast array of fruits, vegetables, grains, seeds, nuts, fiber for cloth, wood for building, and, of course, medicine. From the ancient roots of herbal medicine, the modern sciences of botany, pharmacy, chemistry, and perfumery grew.

Contrary to what many people believe, our ancestors were quite skilled at using natural medicines to prevent and treat disease. Their wisdom has eased the pain and suffering of countless millions from ancient times to the present. Willow was used for the relief of pain and fever in Egypt and North America more than 2,000 years ago, while meadowsweet was widely used in Europe for similar purposes. These salicin-rich plants gave birth to aspirin, the very name being derived from the old botanical name for meadowsweet, *Spirea ulmaria*. Aspirin remains one of the most widely used over-the-counter pain relievers in the world.

The indigenous peoples living in the Andes Mountains of South America used a tree bark to treat fever. The Spanish took the "Peruvian bark" back to Europe where it was used to treat the malaria that was endemic in Rome, having killed commoners and popes alike. In 1820, chemists isolated quinine, the active constituent in the bark, allowing the exploration of the African continent by Europeans, who had died in high numbers due to malaria and yellow fever. During WWII, the Germans and Japanese controlled most of the world's quinine supply, and over 60,000 U.S. troops died from malaria. Scientists have also found that artemisinin, a compound in *Artemisia annua,* is one of the most powerful agents ever discovered for treating the disease. The Chinese have been using this herb to treat malarial fevers for more than 16 centuries.

I love teaching young physicians about the role herbal medicine played and continues to play in modern medicine, having aroused the curiosity of scientists around the world. Although the amount of research dollars pales in comparison to that spent on pharmaceuticals, every day we learn how plants can positively affect our health. Multiple clinical trials have shown that the beautiful hibiscus lowers mild elevations in blood pressure. Ginger alleviates morning sickness, and the most effective treatment to date for irritable bowel syndrome is enteric-coated peppermint oil. More than 40 studies show that St. John's wort is as effective as prescription drugs for alleviating mild forms of depression. Chamomile was shown to reduce anxiety in a study by the University of Pennsylvania. The American Academy of Neurology and the American Headache Society now endorse butterbur as a top-line remedy for preventing migraine headaches. These herbal medicines not only work but they also have a better safety profile and are less expensive than most of their pharmaceutical alternatives.

Herbal medicines can fill a role where pharmaceutical equivalents do not exist. A classic example is milk thistle, an herb known for centuries to be a liver protectant. Now there is scientific proof. Numerous scientific studies show that milk thistle can prevent damage to the liver caused by environmental toxins, alcohol, and medications such as acetaminophen. A study done at Columbia University evaluated children who, while being treated for acute lymphoblastic leukemia (ALL), developed a serious form of liver toxicity brought on by chemotherapy. Half of the kids were given milk thistle; the other half was simply observed. The group treated with milk thistle was able to continue their course of treatment on schedule. Their liver enzymes (an indicator of liver function), even though they were getting chemotherapy, trended back toward the normal range. Milk thistle protected the liver from harm and did not interfere with the effectiveness of the chemotherapy. To date, we have no pharmaceutical that can do that.

From ancient tradition to modern science, there is an abundance of evidence that herbal medicines can be used to improve our well-being. It is also clear that we must use them intelligently. Health is a continuum. On one end is a vibrant and resilient human being and at the other is one who is very ill or near death. In between is a gray area where common sense should dictate our course. There is a time and place for the strong hand of modern medicine. Serious illnesses and injuries are when the risk/benefit almost always tilts in the favor or pharmaceuticals, surgery, and hospitalization. I say risk/benefit intentionally. We should be willing to use more potent and potentially dangerous interventions when the risk of not using them could mean disability, harm, or death. But when the condition is mild and the risk is not great, problems can and do arise when we interfere with the natural processes of the body.

Using milder treatments to treat many of our everyday health problems should be our first choice. The body is well designed for self-healing. Most of the time, all it needs is support as it tries to restore its equilibrium. Hippocrates believed that a physician's primary role was to remove any obstacles that impeded the body's natural ability to get better. I agree. Many of the obstacles getting in the way of health today are poor diet, lack of exercise, unhealthy relationships, chronic stress, and an under-fed spiritual life. Illness is always best treated before it begins. Being healthy is our birthright, and it is also our responsibility.

The first step toward empowerment is knowledge, and that is why I have written this book. You CAN take care of the major-ity of common health problems at home with simple, gentle, and effective treatments. Herbal medicines are woven through-out this book because I believe in their health-giving benefits. I have chosen to emphasize gentle and commonly available herbs because I believe there are plenty of "heroic" medicines in the world already. The recipes provided are those I've used myself, with my own family and with thousands of patients over the years. I pray that they will be of use to you and your family, as well. I will close with one of my favorite quotes:

"Until man duplicates a blade of grass,
nature can laugh at his so-called scientific knowledge.
Remedies from chemicals will never stand in favor
compared with the products of nature,
the living cell of the plant,
the final result of the rays of the sun,
the mother of all life."

Thomas A. Edison

Chapter 9

The Eighteen Essentials

Natural Remedies Every Home Should Have on Hand

S ome herbal medicines, like the infusions and decoctions for example, must be made when needed. They are perishable, their medicinal value is at its peak just when they are made, and they cannot be stored for long.

But other important natural remedies can be made at home and stored for the times when you need them. Here is a list, with recipes, of the 18 preparations I recommend you make ahead of time and store in your pantry to always have on hand.

Tinctures
- Arnica Tincture
- Barberry or Oregon Grape Root Tincture
- Cramp Bark Tincture
- Echinacea Tincture
- Grindelia Compound Tincture
- Herbal Bitter Aperitif

- Licorice Relief Tincture
- Uva Ursi–Corn Silk Tincture
- Witch Hazel Tincture

Glycerites
- German Chamomile Glycerite
- Echinacea Glycerite

Oils
- Calendula Flower Oil
- Mullein Flower Ear Oil
- St. John's Wort Oil

Medicinal Honeys
- Thyme Honey
- Sage Honey

Topical Preparations
- Oatmeal Relief
- Natural Anti-Inflammatory Cream

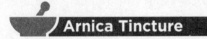

Arnica Tincture

For sprains, strains, and bruises

This should be a first aid remedy in all households. We use a lot of arnica tincture on the ranch. It can be mixed with clay for bug bites or used as a compress for strains and sprains. I even rub it on my mare's tendons after a long ride. Remember to keep it out of reach of children! Some folks can be sensitive to arnica when applied topically—discontinue if it causes a rash.

25 grams *Arnica montana* flowers
125 milliliters menstruum, 40 to 50 percent alcohol

Grind arnica flowers to a coarse powder and put them in a wide-mouthed jar. Add vodka. Stir to make sure that the spoon moves freely. If necessary, add another 25 milliliters of vodka. Put a lid on tightly and shake daily for 2 to 4 weeks. Strain the contents of the jar through muslin cloth. Store the liquid in a dark glass bottle. Label: EXTERNAL USE ONLY. Compost the remaining herb.

How to Use: Put 30 milliliters of tincture in 300 milliliters of water and apply as a compress to sprains, strains, painful spider bites, or any acute injury where there is pain and swelling. It should not be used on open wounds, however, as it is only for topical use.

Barberry or Oregon Grape Root Tincture

For minor wounds and infections

Barberry and Oregon grape root are highly reliable and effective antimicrobial agents against a broad range of bacteria, protozoa, and amoeba. They have both been a mainstay in my practice for decades. I've used them internally to treat diarrhea and other gastrointestinal (GI) infections, as an antiseptic for wounds, gargle for infected gums, douche for vaginal yeast infections, and more.

25 grams barberry or Oregon grape root bark, dried
125 milliliters menstruum, 40 to 50 percent alcohol

Grind or chop the barberry root bark into very small pieces and put in a canning jar. Add 125 milliliters of vodka (80 to 100 proof). Stir. If you need more liquid, add an additional 25 milliliters of vodka. Put on a lid and shake daily for 2 to 4 weeks. Strain. Put the liquid in a dark tincture bottle and label.

How to Use: Adults can take 3 milliliters 3 times a day for acute infection. Use 30 milliliters in 300 milliliters of water as a wash for cuts and wounds.

Note: Berberine-containing herbs should not be used while pregnant or breast-feeding.

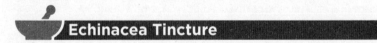

Cramp Bark Tincture

For menstrual cramps, leg cramps, and muscle spasms

Cramp bark is one of my favorite herbs for relieving painful menstrual cramps, leg cramps, and muscle spasms of the back. It relaxes muscles gently but effectively. The trick is taking small frequent doses.

25 grams black haw or cramp bark
125 milliliters vodka (80 to 100 proof)

Grind the herb and put the grinds in a jar. Add the vodka. Put a lid on tightly. Let steep for 2 to 4 weeks. Strain and put the liquid in a dark-colored jar. Label and store in a dark cabinet.

How to Use: Take $1/2$ teaspoon of tincture every 2 to 3 hours, as needed for menstrual cramps. For leg cramps, take 1 teaspoon of tincture an hour before bed.

Note: If you have had a history of calcium oxalate kidney stones, use cramp bark instead of black haw. *If you are pregnant, always discuss the use of black haw, cramp bark, or any herb with your midwife or doctor before using.*

Echinacea Tincture

For colds and coughs and topically for minor wounds

Echinacea was held in high esteem by many indigenous North American peoples for the treatment of fever, cough, sore throat, infections, wounds, and venomous bites. Although it isn't a "cure" for the common cold, it's the closest thing I've found to getting better faster. I've never found echinacea capsules very effective; the tincture and tea work best.

50 grams *Echinacea purpurea* herb or *E. angustifolia* root, dried
250 milliliters solvent, 40 to 60 percent alcohol

Grind the herb to a coarse powder and put the grounds in a widemouthed jar. Add 80-proof vodka or brandy if you want less alcohol. If you want a stronger tincture, use 60 percent alcohol. In this case, you'd multiply 250 (milliliters) x 0.6 (60 percent), which equals 150. That means you would use 150 milliliters of grain alcohol and 100 milliliters of water. I've made them both ways and find they both get the job done. Put a lid on tightly and shake daily for 2 to 4 weeks. Strain the contents of the jar through muslin cloth. Store the liquid in a dark glass bottle. Label. Compost the remaining herb.

How to Use: At the first sign of a cold or upper respiratory infection, adults should take 5 milliliters of the tincture every 4 hours (4 times a day) for 2 to 4 days, as needed. You will find more flavorful versions in Chapter 3.

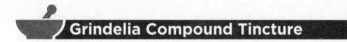

Grindelia Compound Tincture

For cough, postnasal drip, and congestion

Commonly referred to as gumweed, grindelia was widely used by Native Americans to treat bronchial problems and is still recognized for this by the German health authorities. It is one of my go-to herbs for upper respiratory infections with cough, congestion, and postnasal drip. Yerba santa, or holy herb, coats and soothes a sore throat while gently loosening phlegm, making it easier to expectorate. Horehound has been used for many centuries to open the bronchioles and ease children's croupy cough. Licorice remains one of our best medicines for soothing an irritated throat and cough. It is still found in many popular cough and cold medicines. Put them all together and you have a fabulous cold and cough remedy. One of my absolute favorites!

10 grams grindelia flowering tops
5 grams horehound herb
5 grams licorice root
5 grams yerba santa leaves
125 milliliters solvent, 70 percent

Grind herbs in a coffee grinder and put in a widemouthed glass jar. Pour 85 milliliters of grain alcohol and 40 milliliters of water over the herbs. Make sure you can move a spoon easily through the liquid. If you need more liquid, add 15 milliliters grain alcohol and 10 milliliters water. Put a lid on tightly and let steep for 2 weeks, shaking daily. Strain liquid through a muslin cloth and pour the decanted liquid into a dark amber bottle. Put a lid on tightly and label. Compost the leftover herb matter.

Your tincture is ready to be used to make syrup at any time.

To make the syrup: Simply warm 4 ounces of raw honey in a double boiler. Add 40 milliliters of the tincture to the honey, cover, and heat for 10 minutes on the lowest setting. Place in a jar. Take 1 teaspoon every 2 to 4 hours as needed. Amazingly effective!

Note: *This recipe contains licorice, but in a very small amount. It is quite safe when used in the amount recommended for 4 to 6 weeks. But if you have high blood pressure and are concerned, you can remove it from the recipe and increase the horehound to 10 grams.*

Herbal Bitter Aperitif

For gas and bloating, and to enhance overall digestive health

Aperitifs are taken before meals to stimulate the appetite and prepare the GI tract. I've used the following formula for more than 30 years in my practice.

10 grams dandelion root, dried and cut
10 grams gentian root, dried and cut
10 grams chamomile flowers, dried
5 grams Oregon grape root, dried and cut
5 grams fennel seeds
200 milliliters brandy or vodka OR
225 milliliters vegetable glycerin plus 95 milliliters distilled water

Grind the herbs to a coarse powder in an electric coffee grinder. Put the ground herbs into a jar and add liquid. You can make this with brandy or you can make it alcohol free with vegetable glycerin and water. Secure the lid, label, and let sit for 14 days. Make sure you can move the spoon freely through the ingredients. If you need to add more alcohol, add another 40 milliliters brandy or vodka. If you used vegetable glycerin, add another 30 milliliters vegetable glycerin and 10 milliliters water. Shake every day. Strain and put in a clean jar. Label. Compost the herbs.

How to Use: Put 1 teaspoon in $\frac{1}{2}$ cup water (still or carbonated) and drink 15 to 20 minutes before your largest meal of the day, if you used brandy or vodka, or take 2 teaspoons right off the spoon if you made it with glycerin.

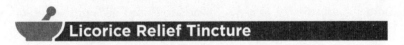

Licorice Relief Tincture

For topical treatment of cold sores and inflammation

25 grams licorice root, cut
125 milliliters vodka (80 proof)

Grind licorice to a coarse powder and put in a jar. Add vodka. Stir. The liquid should completely cover the herb, and your spoon should be able to move freely. If you need more liquid, add an additional 25 milliliters of vodka, put on a lid, and shake daily for 14 days. Strain. Pour the liquid into a dark tincture bottle and label.

How to Use: Insert a clean cotton swab into the tincture and apply to the herpes (cold sore) outbreak. Reapply using a clean cotton swab every hour, while awake, during the first 24 to 48 hours. If applied frequently, it works like magic—there's no other word for it. There are no safety concerns with this topical use of licorice.

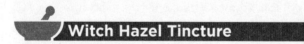

Uva Ursi-Corn Silk Tincture

For minor urinary tract infections

There is nothing that works better for minor, uncomplicated bladder infections than a combination of uva ursi and corn silk. Uva ursi helps fight off the infection, and corn silk soothes and relieves the irritation.

25 grams uva ursi leaf
15 grams corn silk
200 milliliters vodka (80 to 100 proof)

Grind uva ursi and corn silk and put in a jar. Cover with the alcohol. If necessary, add another 40 milliliters vodka to ensure your spoon moves readily through the mixture. Let it sit, covered, and shake daily for 14 days. Strain. Pour into dark bottle, label, and store.

How to Use: Take 3 milliliters in $\frac{1}{4}$ cup water or juice every 2 to 3 hours (up to 6 doses) during first 48 hours of symptoms. Then 3 times per day for 72 hours.

Note: Uva ursi should not be taken longer than 4 weeks and should not be used by pregnant or breast-feeding women.

Witch Hazel Tincture

For topical use on bites, rashes, and hemorrhoids

Trust me, your own homemade witch hazel tincture will far surpass anything you find on a pharmacy shelf. That's because distilled witch hazel has no tannin, and that's what gives the herb its fabulous astringent and medicinal benefits.

50 grams witch hazel bark *(Hamamelis virginiana)*
250 milliliters solvent, 20 percent

Grind the herb and put the grounds in a canning jar. To get 20 percent alcohol strength, just multiply 250 (milliliters) x 0.2 (20 percent), which equals 50. Pour 50 milliliters grain alcohol over the herb and 200 milliliters water. Put a lid on tightly and shake daily for 2 to 4 weeks. Strain the contents of the jar through muslin cloth. Squeeze tightly to remove as much liquid as possible. Store the liquid in a dark glass bottle. Label.

How to Use: You can use witch hazel tincture on insect bites, skin rashes, and hemorrhoids. Just apply the tincture with a cotton ball several times throughout the day.

German Chamomile Glycerite

For upset stomach, colic, anxiousness, and insomnia

In today's crazy, chaotic world, I think many of us could benefit from the use of this gentle herb. Researchers at the University of Pennsylvania found it was highly effective for relieving anxiety, while a study at the University of Michigan found that chamomile helps participants fall asleep faster and wake up fewer times at night compared to those who were given a placebo. You will see that I use chamomile in many recipes throughout this book.

50 grams German chamomile flowers
280 milliliters vegetable glycerin
120 milliliters water

Purchase high-quality chamomile flowers and grind them in your coffee grinder. Place the ground herb in a widemouthed jar and cover with vegetable glycerin and water. Replace the lid. If you need to add more liquid, add an additional 35 milliliters vegetable glycerin and 15 milliliters water. Shake daily for 2 to 4 weeks. Gently heat glycerite in a water bath and then pour the contents of the jar into fine cheesecloth and strain, squeezing firmly to remove liquid. Compost the herbs. Pour liquid into a dark glass bottle and label. The glycerite will keep for 2 years.

How to Use: Take 1 drop per pound of bodyweight up to 60 pounds and then 1 teaspoon for children 60 to 100 pounds, up to 4 times a day, as needed. Teens and adults can take 1 tablespoon up to 4 times a day, as needed.

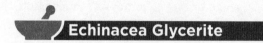

Echinacea Glycerite

For cold, cough, and sore throat

I've had a long and enduring relationship with echinacea and have relied upon it heavily for minor colds, sore throats, and congestion. I prefer to use the glycerite for children, or for adults who cannot tolerate alcohol. The taste is mild and sweet.

50 grams echinacea herb or root
280 milliliters vegetable glycerin
120 milliliters water

Purchase high-quality echinacea herb and/or root and grind in your coffee grinder. Place the ground herb in a widemouthed jar and cover with vegetable glycerin and water. Replace the lid. If you need to add more liquid, add another 35 milliliters vegetable glycerin and 15 milliliters water. Shake daily for 2 to 4 weeks. Gently heat glycerite in a water bath and then pour the contents of the jar into fine cheesecloth and strain.

How to Use: Children for up to 5 days:

15 to 25 pounds: $1/2$ teaspoon every 2 to 3 hours
25 to 50 pounds: $3/4$ teaspoon every 2 to 3 hours
50 to 75 pounds: $1 1/2$ teaspoon every 2 to 3 hours
75 to 100 pounds: 1 teaspoons every 2 to 3 hours
100 to 150 pounds: 2 teaspoons every 2 to 3 hours

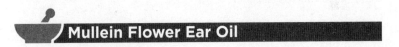

Calendula Flower Oil

For soothing, moisturizing, and cleansing the skin

I grow calendula in my garden, not only for the beauty of its warm orange blossoms, but also because it is my go-to herb for minor skin problems. Calendula is an edible flower, meaning it's OK to use on chafed and sore nipples when nursing. Calendula is wonderful baby oil—much better than many commercial products that contain preservatives and/or mineral oil. Massage a thin layer of oil after bathing. It seals in moisture, has mild antibacterial activity to help prevent secondary infections, and reduces itching.

Calendula flowers, dried or freshly dried
Olive, grape seed, or sunflower seed oil (carrier oil)

Fill a jar $^2/_3$ full with calendula flowers and then cover with the carrier oil. Put on a lid so that it fits tightly. Let it steep in a paper bag in a warm place for 2 to 4 weeks. Strain, bottle, label, and store the oil in a cool dark place.

How to Use: Apply to affected area as needed, 1 to 4 times a day.

Mullein Flower Ear Oil

For minor earache relief

Mullein flowers
Extra-virgin olive oil

Whenever possible, harvest fresh mullein flowers in late summer. Let them sit overnight to remove some of the moisture. Place them in a glass jar and completely cover them with olive oil. If you don't have access to fresh mullein, you can use dried mullein flowers. Make sure the oil is roughly 1 inch higher than the flowers. Place the jar in a brown paper bag, put in a warm sunny place, and let it sit for 2 to 4 weeks. Strain. Put the liquid into a dark bottle, label, and store for up to 1 year.

How to Use: Lie on side with affected ear facing up. Put 2 to 3 drops directly into the ear canal and then gently push and pull the outer ear to work the oil down into the canal. Lie in this position for about 5 minutes. You can put a small ball of cotton in the ear to keep the oil in the ear canal. Repeat this procedure 2 to 3 times a day. *Never put oil in the ear if you see drainage or suspect that the eardrum has ruptured.*

St. John's Wort Oil

For the topical relief of sore muscles, nerve pain, and sunburn

St. John's wort oil is one of my favorite massage oils for relieving sore or overexerted muscles. I have also found it very handy for sunburn (or other burns) and when applied topically for postherpetic neuralgia, or the pain that can linger after the outbreak of shingles.

St. John's wort herb
Extra-virgin olive oil

Whenever possible, harvest fresh St. John's wort herb in flower. Let it sit overnight to remove some of the moisture. If you don't have access to fresh St. John's wort, you can use dried. Place the plant material in a glass jar and completely cover with olive oil. Make sure the oil is roughly 1 inch higher than the flowers. Place the jar in a brown paper bag, put in a warm sunny place, and let it sit for 2 to 4 weeks. Strain. The oil will be a deep ruby red. Beautiful! Put the liquid into a dark bottle, label, and store for up to 1 year.

How to Use: Apply to sore muscles and massage into skin. Can be used in a similar way for postherpetic neuralgia and sunburn. Apply 2 to 3 times per day.

Thyme Honey

Soothes respiratory and skin irritation

One of the most versatile medicinal honeys you can have around the house. Not only is it great for cooking, but you can use it to soothe a cough or apply it topically to a wound. If you have a young child in the house (under 12 months of age) you might want to substitute maple syrup for the honey in the recipe.

$\frac{1}{2}$ cup fresh or $\frac{1}{4}$ cup dried thyme
8 ounces honey

Put honey in saucepan and gently heat. Add the thyme and stir for about 10 minutes. Pour your heated thyme honey into a clean canning jar, put on the lid, and let it sit in a warm place (a windowsill, for example) for 2 to 3 weeks. Using a spatula, scoop out the contents of your jar into a saucepan and gently heat until the honey has become liquid. Using a fine-mesh strainer, pour the honey into a clean jar. Label and store it in a cool, dark cabinet. Your herbal honey will stay good for at least 1 year.

How to Use: For coughs and colds, put 1 teaspoon thyme honey into 1 cup hot water and stir. Add some fresh lemon if desired. You can also just take 1 teaspoon thyme honey straight off the spoon to stop a cough. For wounds, spread a thin layer on a 3 x 3 bandage or gauze and apply. Change daily.

Sage Honey

A strong antiseptic for internal and topical use

Sage honey is another of my kitchen must-haves. Also great for cooking, sage is strongly antiseptic and can be applied topically to a wound or used to ease a sore throat and upper respiratory infection. If you have a young child in the house (under 12 months of age) you might want to substitute maple syrup for the honey in the recipe.

$\frac{1}{2}$ cup fresh or $\frac{1}{4}$ cup dried sage
8 ounces honey

Follow the recipe above, substituting sage herb for the thyme.

How to Use: For coughs and sore throat, take 1 teaspoon sage honey and put in 1 cup hot water and stir. Add some fresh lemon if desired. You could also just take 1 teaspoon sage honey straight off the spoon to relieve a sore throat. For wounds, apply thin layer to a 3 x 3 bandage or gauze and apply. Change daily.

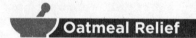

Oatmeal Relief

For itch relief

By using just two common ingredients in your kitchen, you can provide your family with an amazing anti-itch remedy. Use it in the tub to soothe chicken pox, poison ivy, or mosquito bites. Or make it into a paste and apply to a bad bug bite. Totally safe and effective!

4 cups oatmeal, powdered
$\frac{1}{2}$ cup baking soda or cornstarch

Grind the oatmeal into as fine a powder as you can in a blender or electric coffee grinder. Pour the powder into a jar and add baking soda or cornstarch. Mix well. Put on a lid, label, and store in a dark cupboard.

How to Use: This mixture can be made into a paste and applied topically or added to a bath for itch relief. For more nasty rashes, like poison ivy/oak/sumac, I recommend adding a couple table-spoons cool water to $\frac{1}{2}$ cup Oatmeal Relief to make a paste.

Spread a thin coat over the affected area, cover it with plastic wrap or a towel, and let it dry for 30 to 60 minutes. (You don't need the plastic wrap; it just keeps the poultice from falling off and making a mess!) Rinse off the paste with cool or tepid water. Hot water will make you itch. Repeat as often as necessary to relieve itching and inflammation.

For a bath, mix 1 cup Oatmeal Relief into your bathwater. Make sure the bath is warm, not hot. Soak for 20 to 30 minutes. Repeat as necessary.

Note: For those with celiac disease or gluten intolerance, oatmeal can be safely used on the skin.

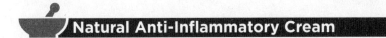

Natural Anti-Inflammatory Cream

To soothe itching, relieve eczema, and heal minor wounds

I prefer to use creams, not salves, oils, or ointments, for red, blistering areas. Creams are a little harder to make, so you may want to purchase an herbal cream made from licorice, calendula, chamomile, and/or other soothing herbs from the local health food store or natural grocer. If you're up for a little adventure, though, you can make this one at home. Unlike steroid creams that can cause thinning of the skin with persistent use, this cream has no adverse effects. It's absolutely amazing for relieving itch, soothing irritated skin, and increasing the skin's natural barrier function.

This recipe requires some prepared ingredients whose recipes you will find elsewhere in the book. Read through the full set of instructions before you begin and follow the steps carefully.

Step 1
3/4 cup (175 milliliters) infused calendula oil OR chamomile oil OR Herbal Sunflower Seed Oil (see recipe, page 210)
2/3 cup coconut oil

2 teaspoons beeswax, grated
6 ounces licorice decoction

Put the first 3 ingredients (infused herbal oil, coconut oil, and beeswax) into a double boiler and gently melt, stirring frequently. When melted, pour into your blender and let cool for about 5 to 10 minutes. It will start to get solid around the edges, but when you shake the blender, it should still be liquid. Use a spatula to scrape the sides to break up any areas that have hardened. Now turn your blender on low; slowly drizzle your licorice decoction into the oil. Use your spatula to scrape down the sides every now and then. Keep drizzling in your licorice until it has all been added.

Step 2
1 teaspoon vitamin E oil
½ teaspoon lavender essential oil

These last two ingredients are optional, but they are both healing and soothing to the skin. If you choose to use them, add them to the cream last, gently mixing them into the cream with your spatula.

Step 3
Pour the cream into jar(s) and store in your refrigerator. Vitamin E prevents the oils from going rancid, and the essential oil keeps down microbial growth. Other than those two ingredients, this cream has no actual preservatives. It will keep for 6 months if stored in the fridge, or about 3 months if kept in the kitchen cupboard.

How to Use: Apply to the affected areas 3 to 4 times a day, as needed.

Stocking the Pantry

I've always been a self-reliant person, and I believe in being prepared. Who wants to wonder if you have the medicine you need when someone in your family gets sick in the middle of the night? Having the remedies and tools you need, when you need them, makes life that much simpler and far less stressful. Every family should have a designated shelf in a cabinet where all first aid supplies are kept, and everyone of a responsible age should know the basics for how to care for minor ailments.

By the time my children were 10 or 11 years old, they knew how to use a thermometer, when and how to use echinacea, make a saltwater gargle, clean and dress a wound, and prepare ginger tea for an upset stomach. Sounds simple and straightforward, doesn't it? Yes, but not for a lot of people. My children tell me that when their college-aged friends come down with diarrhea or a sore throat, they're straight off to urgent care. Not only does this drive up health care costs, it often exposes you to unnecessary diagnostic tests and medications.

Determining what you need to stock in your home pharmacy will take some time and consideration on your part. I have provided step-by-step instructions for making your own natural medicines at home. Now you have to decide what conditions you're most likely to encounter in your own household. Do you have children at home? How easy is it to get to a pharmacy, natural grocer, health food store, and supermarket? What is your budget?

My children are grown now, so remedies for colic or middle ear infections are low on my list, but supplies for wound care, rashes, bug bites, nausea, diarrhea, colds, fever, infection, pain, and stomach troubles are important to keep on hand. We have a little general store about 15 minutes from our cabin, but we are a good 45 minutes from a pharmacy or grocery store, that is if the weather is good. I keep a well-stocked but strategic set of supplies to meet the needs of my family and our critters. We also keep a small first aid kit in the car, and carry one with us when we take long trail rides with the horses. The following suggested list is for your home, so I am assuming that you have clean water, blankets, and so on.

The Durable Basics

These items will last many years if stored in an appropriate moisture-free container. A toolbox, fishing tackle box, or just a decent-sized plastic storage container works well. The main thing you have to monitor is replacing the stock once it's used up.

- Digital thermometer—for checking and monitoring fever
- Tweezers—for removing splinters, stingers, and ticks
- Scissors—to cut bandages and tape
- Box of adhesive bandages (assorted sizes)—to dress minor wounds
- Adhesive strips (butterfly bandages)—for closing wounds
- Box of nonadherent pads (various sizes)—for burns
- Box of sterile gauze pads (3 x 3 inches)—to stop bleeding and dress minor wounds
- Box of sterile gauze pads (4 x 4 inches)—to stop bleeding and dress minor wounds
- Two absorbent compress dressings (5 x 9 inches)—to stop and control bleeding

- Compression wrap bandages (2 and 3 inches wide)—for sprains
- One roller gauze bandage (3 inches wide)—for dressing wounds
- One adhesive cloth tape (10 yards x 1 inch)—for dressing wounds
- Triangular bandage—to immobilize fractures or dislocations
- Cotton balls—for eardrops and to apply tincture
- Rubbing alcohol—for disinfecting and outer ear rinse
- Nonlatex gloves (three to four large pairs)—for protection when working with body fluids
- Antibacterial soap—for cleaning wound area and hands
- 60-milliliter syringe or squeeze bottle—for irrigating wounds

Basic Medications

You'll want to keep these in relatively small supplies and check periodically for expiration dates. Generics work fine and are far less expensive. Obviously, if you don't have young children in the house, you can omit the children's medications from your kit:

- Acetaminophen (325-milligram tab/cap)—for minor pain and fever
- Acetaminophen (children's)—for minor pain and fever
- Diphenhydramine (25-milligram tab/cap)—for minor allergic reactions
- Diphenhydramine (children's)—for minor allergic reactions
- Aspirin (81-milligram) chewable—for chest pain, analgesia
- Ibuprofen (200-milligram tab/cap)—for minor pain and fever
- Eyedrops—to assist in removing foreign matter from the eye
- Probiotics (shelf stable; *Lactobacillus* GG and/or *Saccharomyces boulardii*)—for diarrhea, IBS, and to take if on antibiotics
- DGL (deglycyrrhizinated licorice)—for heartburn
- Vitamin C (100- to 250-milligram tablets)—for colds, minor infections

- Zinc lozenges (5- to 10-milligram zinc gluconate or glycinate per lozenge)—colds, upper respiratory infections
- Butterbur standardized extract—for allergies and migraine prevention

Kitchen Items

For making natural medicines at home, you'll need some basic kitchen equipment and supplies, many of which you probably already have:

- Measuring spoons and cups—for measuring your ingredients
- Wooden spoon and plastic spatula—for stirring and blending
- Knife and cutting board—for chopping herbs
- Cheese grater—inexpensive, handheld grater for beeswax
- Funnels of different sizes—for pouring liquids into bottles
- Tea/coffee mugs—for drinking all your wonderful herbal teas
- Tea ball or tea strainer—convenient for small batches of infusions/decoctions
- Large strainer—for straining larger batches of tinctures, oils, and honeys
- Cotton or muslin cloths—for pressing tinctures and oils
- Large mixing bowls of various sizes—for holding strained liquids
- Ice cube tray—for making medicinal ice cubes
- Kitchen scale—basic scale that can measure grams and ounces
- Kitchen blender—basic electric blender works fine; Vitamix works awesome
- Electric coffee grinder—for grinding herbs; keep one dedicated to herb work
- Double boiler—really a must-have to prevent scorching oils and salves
- Saucepans with lids; glass/stainless steel preferred—for making decoctions and salves

- Widemouthed quart canning jars—for making tinctures, oils, and honeys
- Dark glass bottles, some with eyedroppers—for finished tinctures
- Small jars or tins—for salves and ointments
- Labels for jars—so you know what's what
- Electric cooking pot (like a Crock-Pot, though optional)—if you have a double boiler, you don't need this

Cupboard Items

When possible, purchase oils that are organic and/or expeller pressed. Have the following on hand:

- 16 ounces almond, grape seed, or sesame oil
- 16 ounces coconut oil
- 16 ounces sunflower seed oil
- 16 ounces olive oil
- 1-pound box baking soda
- 1-pound box cornstarch
- 1-pound salt, noniodized, not sea salt (for nasal irrigation)
- 1 quart honey, raw
- 1 jar maple syrup
- 1 box oatmeal, instant or steel cut
- 1 quart apple cider vinegar, organic
- 1 pint white vinegar
- Lemon juice
- Onions and garlic

Essential Oils

Purchase these in dark amber bottles (0.5 to 1.0 fluid ounce):

- Eucalyptus
- Lavender
- Oregano

- Peppermint
- Tea tree
- Thyme

Herbs

I have provided the botanical name for each of these herbs so you can ensure you are purchasing the correct genus and species. These are recommended amounts; you may need more or less depending upon your household. Some of these herbs, such as calendula, peppermint, sage, skullcap, and thyme, can be easily grown in your garden or in pots on your porch, and you can make your medicines out of the fresh plant:

- 4 ounces arnica flowers *(Arnica montana)*
- 4 ounces barberry root bark *(Berberis vulgaris)* OR Oregon grape root bark *(Mahonia aquifolium, Berberis aquifolium)*
- 4 ounces calendula flowers *(Calendula officinalis)*
- 4 ounces chamomile flowers *(Matricaria recutita)*
- 1 ounce cinnamon powder *(Cinnamomum zeylanicum, C. verum, Cassia cinnamomum)*
- 2 ounces corn silk *(Zea mays)*
- 2 ounces cramp bark *(Viburnum opulus)* or black haw bark *(Viburnum prunifolium)*
- 2 ounces dandelion root *(Taraxacum officinale)*
- 4 ounces echinacea root *(Echinacea purpurea, E. angustifolia)*
- 1 ounce elderflowers *(Sambucus nigra)*
- 2 ounces fennel seed *(Foeniculum vulgare)*
- 1 ounce ginger rhizome *(Zingiber officinale)*
- 1 ounce grindelia flowering tops *(Grindelia robusta, G. camporum)*
- 1 ounce horehound herb *(Marrubium vulgare)*
- 1 ounce lemon balm herb *(Melissa officinalis)*

- 4 ounces licorice root *(Glycyrrhiza glabra)*
- 1 ounce nettle leaf *(Urtica dioica)*
- 2 ounces peppermint leaves *(Mentha x piperita)*
- 2 ounces raspberry leaves *(Rubus idaeus)*
- 2 ounces sage leaves *(Salvia officinalis)*
- 2 ounces skullcap herb *(Scutellaria lateriflora)*
- 2 ounces St. John's wort herb *(Hypericum perforatum)*
- 2 ounces thyme herb *(Thymus vulgaris)*
- 4 ounces uva ursi leaves *(Arctostaphylos uva ursi)*
- 2 ounces yarrow flowering tops *(Achillea millefolium)*
- 1 ounce yerba santa leaves *(Eriodictyon californicum)*
- 4 ounces witch hazel bark *(Hamamelis virginiana)*

Odds and Ends

- 6 ounces beeswax—for salves and creams
- 6 ounces bentonite or French green clay—for insect bites
- Neti pot or neti bottle—for nasal irrigation
- Bulb syringe—for infant nasal irrigation
- 1 quart vegetable glycerin—for making alcohol-free tinctures
- 1 liter grain alcohol (190 proof)—for tincture making
- 1 liter vodka and/or brandy (80 to 100 proof)—for tincture making
- 1 ounce vitamin E oil (d-alpha tocopherol)—antioxidant for creams, oils, and salves

Resources

You will be able to find many of your ingredients at local grocery stores, pharmacies, natural grocers, and health food/herb shops. You can pick up grain alcohol and vodka at any store where alcohol is sold. If you're lucky enough to have a nearby hobby or fabric shop, you can pick up muslin or cotton pressing cloths really cheap. Farmer's markets and local beekeepers are great resources for raw honey and beeswax. There isn't much you cannot find on Amazon. I have included some additional resources. I am a price-comparison shopper. I want good quality at a good price. Many vendors that sell online offer free shipping.

The one area where I am super-picky is when it comes to purchasing herb seeds and bulk herbs for medicine making. I trust the following resources I've listed. I know that I am getting the correct genus and species and the herb is of high quality. Your medicine will only be as good as the raw material you start with!

The Container Store
www.containerstore.com
For dark bottles, salve containers, and canning jars

eBeeHoney
www.ebeehoney.com
This source is a nice place to purchase honey and high-quality beeswax. Check for sources of locally grown honey, as well.

Essential Depot
www.essentialdepot.com
This vendor sells USP-grade kosher vegetable glycerin at good prices.

Frontier Natural Products Co-op
www.frontiercoop.com
Here is wonderful one-stop shopping for wildcrafted and organic herbs, vegetable glycerin, natural flavorings, green clay, beeswax, and other supplies.

Horizon Herbs
www.horizonherbs.com
This is a great place for purchasing organic and medicinal herb seeds.

Mountain Rose Herbs
www.mountainroseherbs.com
Here's my go-to source for high-quality wildcrafted and USDA-certified organic herbs for medicine making.

Rich Gulch Products
http://blitz.goldrush.com/mathrespresses/order.htm
If you want to purchase a reasonably priced herbal tincture press, this is the best source.

Herbs for Today

A Modern Materia Medica

This section is a brief summary of the most important herbs discussed in this book, and is intended to provide background for my recommendations. It is not an exhaustive review of the scientific or historic evidence. References may be found at *drlowdog.com*.

Arnica flowers (*Arnica montana*)

Use: Arnica flowers have been used for centuries for the topical relief of bruises, strains, sprains, and swelling. The German health authorities recognize arnica flowers for the external treatment of "injury and for consequences of accidents, e.g., hematoma, dislocations, contusions, edema due to fracture, rheumatic muscle and joint problems, inflammation of the oral and throat region and inflammation caused by insect bites." A study of 204 people with osteoarthritis found that arnica gel and ibuprofen gel were equally effective for relieving pain when applied to the hands for three weeks. Another study found arnica gel to be beneficial in patients with osteoarthritis of the knees. Studies have shown that the flowers contain substances that are highly effective for relieving inflammation and pain.

Safety: Arnica is considered safe when used externally on unbroken skin. Long-term topical use can cause irritation and an eczema-like rash. Arnica should not be used topically for longer than 10 to 14 days. Arnica should not be taken internally! Animal studies show that internal use can cause shortness of breath, elevation of blood pressure, heart damage, and death in overdose. Homeopathic arnica preparations may be taken internally.

Barberry root bark *(Berberis vulgaris)*

Use: Barberry plants have been used medicinally for at least 2,500 years. The herb is still used in India and the Middle East to treat gallbladder and digestive disorders, heartburn, and infection. Barberry contains a number of alkaloids, the principal one being berberine, which is also present in goldenseal, Oregon grape root, and others. Berberine is available as a pharmaceutical drug in some countries and as a dietary supplement in the United States. Berberine has been shown to exert a number of actions including antimicrobial, anti-inflammatory, and astringent. For a more detailed discussion of berberine, see the entry on Oregon grape root.

Safety: All berberine-containing plants are contraindicated for internal use during pregnancy and breast-feeding.

Black haw bark *(Viburnum prunifolium)* and cramp bark *(Viburnum opulus)*

Use: Black haw bark was used by indigenous women to prevent miscarriage and slow uterine bleeding. Physicians of the 19th century valued black haw as a uterine tonic and for the prevention of miscarriage. King's American Dispensatory, one of the leading Eclectic medical texts of the time, states that black haw "acts promptly in spasmodic dysmenorrhea, especially with excessive flow." It was officially listed in the 1882 *United States Pharmacopoeia* and is still considered almost specific for cramps in the legs, especially when occurring at night. The condition for which black haw is most valued is threatened abortion. Today, both European and American herbalists recommend black haw for painful menstrual cramps, threatened miscarriage, leg cramps, tension headaches, after-birth pains, and muscle spasm. There have not been any randomized, controlled human clinical trials conducted with *Viburnum prunifolium* to confirm any of the historical uses for this herb. Research has been limited to animal studies.

Safety: There are no contraindications for the use of black haw in pregnancy or breast-feeding. Black haw is given the following restriction in the *Botanical Safety Handbook:* "Individuals with a history of kidney stones should use this herb cautiously." This is due to the presence of oxalates. Cramp bark is considered a safe alternative because it does not contain oxalates. Some books note a risk of interaction with anticoagulant medication. This theoretical risk is most likely based upon the presence of salicin. An individual consuming 1,000 milligrams of black haw would be ingesting roughly 2 milligrams of salicin. (For comparison, a baby aspirin contains 81 milligrams of acetylsalicylic acid.)

Butterbur *(Petasites hybridus)*

Use: Butterbur is a large-leaved plant that was used for centuries in Europe, northern Africa, and Asia to relieve coughs, congestion, and asthma. Scientists have found compounds in the plant that reduce smooth muscle constriction in the lungs and shrink swollen nasal membranes, providing evidence for its historical uses. Several European clinical trials have now shown that butterbur can be as effective as the leading drugs for seasonal allergies. It may be of benefit for those with asthma, as well. A study of 64 adults and 16 children at the Heidelberg University, in

Germany, reported a decrease in the number, duration, and severity of asthma attacks during two months of butterbur therapy compared to baseline. Butterbur extracts are not sedating and are very well tolerated in both kids and adults.

Butterbur is so effective for the prevention of migraine headaches in both children and adults that it is now a first-line recommendation for migraine prophylaxis by the American Academy of Neurology, the American Headache Society, and the Canadian Headache Society.

Safety: Butterbur contains small amounts of pyrrolizidine alkaloids, compounds that can damage the liver over time. Only purchase standardized extracts that say they are FREE of pyrrolizidine alkaloids. Safety in pregnancy is unknown, so butterbur should probably be avoided.

Calendula flowers *(Calendula officinalis)*

Use: In addition to being pretty, pot marigold flowers have been used since ancient times to soothe minor inflammations of the mouth, throat, and esophagus, and topically for skin infections and slow-healing wounds. Many authoritative European health organizations echo the extensive historical reputation of calendula for these conditions. Human studies have shown that calendula extracts help prevent radiation dermatitis in women undergoing treatment for breast cancer. A study in 66 infants found that calendula ointment was highly effective for treating diaper dermatitis (rash) when applied three times a day for ten days. Another study of 34 patients with poorly healing venous leg ulcers found that calendula extract led to a 41 percent improvement in wound closure, versus 14.5 percent in the control group. There's no question that calendula ranks supreme when it comes to soothing irritated and/or damaged skin.

Safety: A final toxicology report from the Cosmetic Ingredient Review Expert Panel concluded that calendula extracts are not irritating, sensitizing, or photosensitizing, and are safe for use in topical preparations and cosmetics. There are no contraindications for calendula in pregnancy or breast-feeding in the *Botanical Safety Handbook* or by the German health authorities.

California poppy herb *(Eschscholzia californica)*

Use: This beautiful poppy is California's state flower and has been used as a food and medicine by Native Americans. The young leaves were boiled and eaten as a vegetable, and the whole upper part of the plant (leaves, flowers, and stem) were used to make teas to relieve tooth pain, headache, and as a mild sedative. Today, herbalists still widely use California poppy as a mild pain reliever, to induce sleep, and to take the edge off those who feel anxious. California poppy is in the same family as opium poppy; however, it does not have the same powerful effects. The only clinical trial conducted in humans that I'm aware of is a study in 2004 of 264 people with generalized anxiety that found the combination of hawthorn, magnesium, and California poppy to be safe and effective. Basic science shows that the herb acts on GABA receptors in the brain, similar to a benzodiazepine without the habit-forming tendency of the drug. I've used this herb for decades and find it to be highly reliable for folks who have difficulty sleeping due to aches, pains, or worry.

Safety: The *Botanical Safety Handbook* states that California poppy should not be used during pregnancy or while breast-feeding.

Chamomile flowers *(Matricaria recutita)*

Use: Chamomile flowers have been used as a medicine since ancient times by peoples all over the world. Two dominant chamomiles are traded on the market. Roman chamomile *(Chamaemelum nobile)* and German chamomile *(Matricaria recutita)*, each having differing chemical compositions. I am only referring to German chamomile in this book. The tasty tea has been used to calm the nerves, ease spasms of the gut, and soothe inflammations of the skin and gastrointestinal tract. Chamomile is recognized by the German health authorities and the European Scientific Cooperative on Phytotherapy for the treatment of gastrointestinal spasms and inflammatory conditions of the skin and oral mucosa.

Chamomile has long been considered a "children's herb," as it is soothing to the tummy and the nerves. Chamomile was studied in babies, roughly three weeks of age, and found safe and effective for relieving infant colic when given in combination with fennel seed and lemon balm. Clinical trials have shown chamomile extracts to be as effective as over-the-counter steroid creams for childhood eczema. The German Commission E monograph lists "inflammations of the skin and mucous membranes and bacterial diseases involving the skin" as approved indications for chamomile.

And chamomile isn't just for babies. A randomized controlled trial found that German chamomile extract was highly effective for relieving anxiety in a study of 57 patients diagnosed with mild to moderate generalized anxiety disorder. This study also showed an improvement in depressive symptoms, as well.

Safety: Chamomile has an amazing safety record that spans the past 25 centuries.

German chamomile is not contraindicated in pregnancy or breast-feeding by any health authority. However, Roman chamomile *should not* be used in pregnancy. Do not use in or around the eyes. A study in humans found that when chamomile tea is used as eyewash, it might induce allergic conjunctivitis. Allergic reactions, although rare, have occurred with both internal and topical use of chamomile.

Cinnamon powder *(Cinnamomum zeylanicum, C. cassia)*
Use: Cinnamon has been treasured for its fragrance, culinary

use, and medicinal effects since ancient times. There is only one "true" or "real" cinnamon and that is *Cinnamomum zeylanicum*, which is from Ceylon, or what is now Sri Lanka. You may also see it sold under the alternative scientific name *Cinnamomum verum*. All other types of cinnamon are collectively referred to as cassia, mostly native to China and Southeast Asia. The vast majority of cinnamon sold in this country is *Cinnamomum cassia*. True cinnamon and cassia share similar properties, such as the ability to inhibit the growth of fungi and yeast, destroy many types of bacteria, relieve nausea, and help regulate blood sugar and lower cholesterol. Cinnamon is an excellent digestive aid, relieving gas and bloating and assisting in the digestion of fats.

Safety: Ceylon cinnamon contains a very low level of coumarin, a substance that can harm the liver when taken in large quantities. However, cassia contains a much higher level. This isn't really a problem in food, but be wary when taking cinnamon supplements for high blood sugar and other conditions. In those cases, I recommend using true cinnamon. During pregnancy, cinnamon should only be used as a culinary spice. Therapeutic or medicinal doses should be avoided.

Corn silk *(Zea mays)*

Use: The dried stigmas and styles of corn were used topically in Maya, Inca, and American traditional medicine to treat bruises, swellings, sores, and rash. Corn silk was held in high esteem for the treatment of acute and chronic bladder infection/inflammation and urethritis. In 1880, the pharmaceutical company Parke-Davis introduced a corn silk product for the treatment of urinary pain and spasm. The *British Herbal Compendium* lists corn silk as both a mild diuretic and urinary demulcent (soothing agent).

Safety: Corn silk is quite benign and is often included in herbal formulae designed to ease the pain of urinary tract infections. No contraindications are known.

Cranberry *(Vaccinium macrocarpon)*

Use: Studies show that cranberries prevent urinary tract infections by inhibiting the ability of bacteria to adhere or attach to the urethra and bladder wall. Various cranberry preparations in clinical studies have been found effective for preventing urinary tract infections in men, women, and children. However, studies using cranberry juice suffer from considerable dropout rates, because it's hard for participants to drink three servings of the juice every day long term. A 12-month study in 150 sexually active women found that both cranberry juice and cranberry tablets significantly decreased the number of symptomatic bladder infections compared with placebo. However, women preferred the tablets, and the cost was less than half that of the juice.

Safety: Cranberry is very safe; however, tablets are better long term, given the calories and sugar in juice. Several case reports describe an interaction between cranberry juice and the blood thinner warfarin (Coumadin); however, clinical pharmacokinetic studies have failed to show any interaction. Cranberry juice and tablets are safe in pregnancy and breast-feeding.

Dandelion root *(Taraxacum officinale)*

Use: "One man's weed is another man's medicine" is certainly true when it comes to dandelion. Dandelion root enhances digestion by gently promoting the secretion of stomach acid, and the release of bile from the gallbladder and enzymes from the pancreas. When used on a regular basis, it improves the digestion of proteins, fats, and starches. And because bile is a natural laxative, dandelion root helps normalize sluggish bowels. It is rich in inulin, a prebiotic that serves to feed and encourage the growth of healthy gut microflora. The root also offers considerable protection to the liver from a variety of toxins. Although I have focused on the root in this text, modern science has confirmed that dandelion leaves act as a gentle and effective diuretic.

Because it does not deplete potassium to the same degree as other diuretics, it is considered to be an optimal solution when a diuretic is occasionally required.

Safety: Those with stomach ulcers should not use dandelion root because its bitter nature can stimulate the production of stomach acid. Although dandelion is considered safe during pregnancy and lactation, caution should be exercised with the use of any diuretic. Rare allergic reactions to dandelion can occur.

Dong quai root *(Angelica sinensis)*

Use: Dong quai has been used in traditional Chinese medicine (TCM) for at least 20 centuries. It is generally regarded as a tonic for those with fatigue or low vitality, or those who are recovering from illness, and is widely used to relieve pelvic pain and regulate the menstrual cycle. The company Merck introduced the herb to the Western world in 1899, under the trade name Eumenol, a product designed to ease menstrual pain. Modern-day studies have confirmed that dong quai has anti-inflammatory, analgesic, and antispasmodic activity. It most specifically benefits women who have menstrual cramping and light menstrual bleeding.

Safety: Dong quai should not be used during pregnancy or while breast-feeding. It should not be used in women with heavy menstrual periods. Some studies suggest that dong quai should not be used in women with breast cancer.

Echinacea root *(Echinacea purpurea, E. angustifolia)*

Use: Echinacea has a strong history as a medicinal agent in North America, and was highly valued by the Kiowa, Cheyenne, and Lakota for sore throat, coughs, wounds, and as an analgesic. It has been extensively studied for the treatment of acute upper respiratory infection (URI). The strongest evidence is for the use of *Echinacea purpurea* in the treatment of URI. A recent review in the journal *American Family Physician* concluded that *E. purpurea* preparations improve cold symptoms in adults. And a recent four-month Canadian study of 755 healthy adults found that *E. purpurea* herb/root extract significantly reduced the number of virally confirmed colds compared to placebo. A randomized study of 500 children ages 2 to 11 years found that the group receiving *E. purpurea* had a 28 percent decreased risk of developing a subsequent URI when compared to placebo. A combination of echinacea, propolis, and vitamin C decreased the number of upper respiratory infections, the duration of symptoms, and the number of days of illness as compared with placebo in a group of 430 children ages 1 to 5 years.

Safety: An extensive review of the safety of echinacea products concluded that, overall, "adverse events are rare, mild, and reversible." Concerns have been raised that echinacea could worsen autoimmune disease, but this is based on theoretical considerations. Allergic reactions, although rare, have been reported, particularly in those with allergies to the daisy family.

Fennel seed *(Foeniculum vulgare)*

Use: Fennel has been used as a medicine, food flavoring, and vegetable since ancient times. Modern science has verified the relaxing effect that fennel exerts upon the digestive tract, and the mucus-thinning, expectorant activity of the seeds. The seeds, either raw or candied, are popular after-dinner condiments for easing gas and bloating in East Indian restaurants. A study of 93 breast-fed babies with colic found that the combination of fennel, chamomile, and lemon balm decreased crying time by more than double compared to babies receiving placebo over a period of a week. The tea or syrup is often given to children for mild upper respiratory infections because fennel can loosen phlegm, making expectoration easier.

Safety: During pregnancy, fennel should be used only as a spice and flavoring. People who are allergic to members of the Apiaceae family (celery, carrots) should use caution when consuming fennel.

Ginger rhizome *(Zingiber officinale)*

Use: Ginger has been highly valued as a spice, flavoring agent, and medicine for centuries. The herb has been used for a variety of conditions, but it is chiefly known as an antiemetic, anti-inflammatory, digestive aid, carminative, and warming agent. Ginger is excellent for relieving intestinal gas, bloating, and spasm. Numerous human studies have demonstrated the effectiveness of dried ginger rhizome/root in relieving morning sickness, motion sickness, and postoperative nausea. Ginger contains anti-inflammatory compounds called *gingerols,* which explains the strong historical use of ginger for improving symptoms of arthritis when consumed regularly. Of course, many people like the warm feeling they get when taking ginger, which can be helpful for those with poor circulation or Raynaud's. Ginger, fresh or dried, can help relieve a sore throat, and studies show it can help fend off cold viruses.

Safety: Do not exceed doses of 1,000 to 1,500 milligrams of dried ginger a day during pregnancy. Doses of greater than 3 grams of dried ginger a day may interact with blood-thinning/anticoagulant medications, and may cause digestive upset and heartburn.

Grindelia flowering tops
(Grindelia camporum, G. robusta)

Use: Grindelia, commonly referred to as gumweed, was widely used by Native Americans to treat bronchial problems as well as skin afflictions of all kinds, including allergic reactions to poison ivy and poison oak plants. Official recognition of the dried leaf and flowering tops of grindelia came with the introduction of the herb in the *United States Pharmacopoeia* from 1882 to about 1926, and then the *National Formulary* from 1926 to 1960. The German health authorities approved grindelia for congestion of the upper respiratory tract. Most herbalists use grindelia when there is significant postnasal drip, cough, and chest congestion. Grindelia was commonly included in asthma formulations, particularly in combination with licorice, due to its antispasmodic effect.

Safety: There is no information available on the safety of grindelia in pregnancy, so I recommend avoiding it.

Hops strobiles *(Humulus lupulus)*

Use: Although hops may be best known for the bitterness it imparts in the brewing of beer, they have long been used to treat excitability and insomnia, improve appetite and digestion, and relieve toothache and nerve pain throughout much of the world.

Today, the German health authorities endorse the use of hops for "discomfort due to restlessness or anxiety and sleep disturbances." Research suggests that part of its sedative action may work in a similar way to melatonin. Three controlled studies have shown that the combination of hops and valerian is more effective than placebo and similar in effectiveness to prescription sleep medication for shortening the time it takes to fall asleep and improving sleep quality.

Long favored by midwives, scientists have identified at least one key compound in hops, 8-prenylnaringenin, with significant estrogenic activity. A six-week study found that a standardized hop extract decreased the number of hot flashes, night sweats, and insomnia in menopausal women.

Safety: Given the potential estrogenic activity of hops, women who've had breast cancer should probably avoid hops until more is known. Safety in pregnancy is not known. Hops may have sedative effects, so one should not drive or operate heavy machinery while using.

Horehound herb *(Marrubium vulgare)*

Use: The woolly leaves and flowering tops of this mint family member have been used as a cough and cold remedy for centuries. Ancient Romans appreciated it as both an expectorant and digestive aid. Its popularity spread to the United States, and it was used medicinally during the colonial period. What's more, it was officially listed in the *United States Pharmacopoeia* from 1860 to 1910. The herb has been used for hundreds of years to ease chronic coughs and wheezing, and was widely used for children's coughs and croup. Many older people still remember horehound cough drops.

The two main compounds in horehound—marrubiin and volatile oils—are believed to be responsible for its expectorant and cough-relieving activity. Marrubiin acts as a mucolytic, allowing thick secretions to be more easily expectorated. The small amount of mucilage present in the plant may ease an irritated cough. It has a bitter taste, which explains its other use as a digestive tonic. The German health authorities approve the use of horehound for gas, bloating, and poor appetite.

Safety: Horehound is not recommended during pregnancy because of possible uterine stimulation.

Lemon balm herb *(Melissa officinalis)*

Use: Once referred to as "the gladdening herb," lemon balm has been treasured for its calming properties for centuries. Avicenna, a revered Islamic physician, prescribed the herb because it "makes the heart merry." Today, lemon balm is very popular for soothing nerves, easing digestive disturbances, and promoting restful sleep. Compounds in the herb have been shown to have a sedative effect, as well as significant antispasmodic activity. Lemon balm, in combination with fennel and chamomile, was shown to be highly effective for relieving colic in three-week-old babies.

In double-blind studies, German researchers have demonstrated lemon balm's ability to ease symptoms of restlessness, excitability, and anxiety. The herb is a wonderful carminative and is often woven into formulations for those whose emotions often affect their gut.

Scientists have identified several compounds in lemon balm that are able to block the herpes simplex 1 virus. Two clinical trials found that lemon balm extract shortens the duration and severity of the herpes outbreak when applied topically three to four times a day.

Safety: Lemon balm is quite gentle and safe being used in the very young and the elderly alike. There are no contraindications in the scientific literature.

Licorice root (*Glycyrrhiza glabra*)

Use: Licorice has been held in high esteem as a medicinal agent since ancient times. The roots have potent anti-inflammatory activity and are widely used for digestive, respiratory, and skin complaints. It has been used to treat and heal stomach and duodenal ulcers for centuries, and was popular for this purpose in conventional medicine until the 1980s. Its limitation long term was its ability to cause the retention of sodium and water, leading to hypertension, and the excretion of potassium, which can be dangerous if not closely monitored. Researchers removed the compound responsible for this adverse effect, and when deglycyrrhizinated licorice (DGL) was given at a dose of 380 milligrams three times a day to 169 patients with chronic duodenal ulcers, it was shown to be as effective as antacid or cimetidine. It remains popular today for this purpose and for the relief of gastroesophageal reflux (GERD).

Licorice has been shown to soothe sore throats, promote thinner mucus and thus ease chest congestion, and relieve cough. It also has significant activity against numerous respiratory viruses. This is why licorice is included in so many modern cough/cold products.

Studies have also shown that when applied topically, licorice can improve skin hydration and reduce inflammation in those with atopic dermatitis. It also can be highly effective for inactivating the herpes virus when applied topically during an outbreak.

Safety: Licorice is contraindicated (except for topical use or short three- to four-day duration) in those with liver disease, kidney disease, high blood pressure, and during pregnancy. The German health authorities limit the long-term use of licorice to no more than 100 milligrams of glycyrrhizin a day. That is roughly 1,000 to 1,200 milligrams a day of licorice root.

Nettle leaf (Urtica dioica)

Use: Nettle has long been valued as a nutritious food source, as well as a diuretic and for the relief of arthritis. The German health authorities approve the use of nettle leaf as supportive therapy for rheumatic ailments and as a diuretic for bladder inflammation and the prevention of kidney stones. They also approve nettle root for difficulty in urination due to enlarged prostate. Who knew the humble stinging nettle had so much to offer? In addition to these traditional uses, nettle leaf is also used for the relief of allergic rhinitis. A randomized trial found that 600 milligrams a day of freeze-dried nettle was more effective than placebo for the majority of symptoms.

Safety: Fresh stinging nettles cause skin irritation and should be handled with care. Raw fresh nettles should not be consumed. Consume only powdered, extracted, or cooked nettle leaf. Nettle leaf is not contraindicated in pregnancy or lactation; however, the safety of nettle root during pregnancy is uncertain at this time.

Oregon grape root bark (Mahonia aquifolium)

Use: Oregon grape is related to barberry (see entry for this herb). The indigenous peoples of the Pacific Northwest relied upon its medicine for centuries to treat skin and gastrointestinal ailments, as well as for fever and infection. Interestingly, modern research has confirmed its historical use for psoriasis.

The root bark is particularly rich in alkaloids, the dominant one being berberine, which has been shown to inhibit many of the bacteria and parasites that can cause intestinal infections, including the diarrhea-producing *Vibrio cholera, Escherichia coli, Giardia lamblia,* and *Entamoeba histolytica.* Clinical trials conducted in India found that berberine improved gastrointestinal symptoms and resulted in a marked reduction in *Giardia*-positive stools. In comparison to metronidazole (Flagyl), another popular giardiasis medication, berberine was nearly as effective at half the dose.

Berberine also has significant antifungal activity against a variety of *Candida* species, making it a highly effective remedy for vaginal yeast infections. Two teaspoons of the root bark are simmered in three cups water for 20 minutes, strained, and allowed to cool. Douche once a day for five days, making the preparation fresh daily.

In addition to the potent antimicrobial activity of the plant, a recent review of human clinical trials evidence concluded that berberine appears to be effective for treating high blood sugar and cholesterol/triglycerides in people with type 2 diabetes, though larger studies are needed to confirm this.

Safety: All berberine-containing plants are contraindicated for internal use during pregnancy and breast-feeding.

Peppermint leaves *(Mentha x piperita)*

Use: Peppermint is one of our most cherished herbal remedies. It relaxes the smooth muscles of the gastrointestinal tract and improves the flow of bile from the gallbladder, helping the body digest fats. This is why peppermint is commonly used to relieve intestinal gas and abdominal cramping. Studies show that enteric-coated peppermint oil capsules are superior to conventional treatments for treating irritable bowel syndrome (IBS), a condition that is characterized by recurring bouts of abdominal pain and constipation, diarrhea, or both. These studies also show that peppermint oil is very well tolerated.

Peppermint and its active constituent, menthol, can thin mucus, help loosen phlegm, and break up a cold. The Food and Drug Administration approves the use of mentholated ointments, lozenges, and steam inhalants for alleviating coughs. When applied to the neck and chest, the medicated vapors quickly relieve coughing. The mild anesthetic and cooling properties of menthol make it ideal for soothing a sore throat.

Peppermint applied topically has a soothing effect upon the skin. It reduces itching caused by bug bites or poison ivy, and relieves minor aches and pains such as muscle cramps, arthritis, and headache.

Safety: Peppermint should not be used if you have GERD, because peppermint can worsen heartburn. Never apply peppermint or mentholated oil to the face of an infant or child under the age of five years, because it may cause spasms that inhibit breathing.

Raspberry leaves *(Rubus idaeus)*

Use: Raspberry leaf has been used as a "family" medicine for centuries. The fruits of the black and red raspberry shrubs were enjoyed as a tasty food, while the leaves were used as an astringent for a variety of conditions, principally diarrhea in children. Raspberry leaf tea has also been used as a uterine tonic for hundreds of years, and it remains a popular pregnancy tea. Many lay herb books promote the use of raspberry leaf for the prevention of miscarriage, to ease morning sickness, and to ensure a timely birth. A survey of 172 certified nurse midwives found that, of the 90 midwives who used herbal preparations,

63 percent recommended red raspberry leaf. A double-blind, placebo-controlled study of 192 low-risk, first-time pregnant women randomized women to take raspberry leaf tablets (1,200 milligrams twice a day) or placebo from 32 weeks gestation until labor. Raspberry leaf was found to cause no adverse effects for the mothers or babies, but contrary to popular belief, did not shorten the first stage of labor. It did, however, shorten the second stage of labor, and there was a lower rate of forceps deliveries in the treatment group.

Safety: There are no contraindications to the use of raspberry leaves.

Sage leaves *(Salvia officinalis)*

Use: The genus name salvia, from the word *salvere,* "to save," was likely given in honor of its place in medicine. The herb is said to clear the mind and improve memory, and the term "sage" is associated with wisdom or being a wise elder. Interestingly, researchers have found that sage essential oil inhibits acetylcholinesterase, the enzyme targeted by many Alzheimer's drugs. Animal studies and small human trials suggest sage may improve mood and cognition in both healthy adults and those with Alzheimer's dementia.

Sage is a useful remedy for sore throats. One clinical trial of 286 people with acute pharyngitis (sore throat) found that a 15 percent sage spray provided symptom relief within two hours of taking the first treatment. Similar results were found when an echinacea/sage spray was compared to a chlorhexadine/lidocaine spray in 154 patients with acute pharyngitis.

The German health authorities endorse the use of sage as a treatment for excessive sweating based on traditional use and small human studies. Sage may have weak estrogenic properties, explaining its effectiveness for relieving night sweats in menopausal women.

Sage is commonly used to aid digestion, stimulate digestive enzymes, and alleviate intestinal cramping. This is one reason it's often cooked with beans or other gas-producing foods. Sage has antibacterial activity, which might also explain its use in gastroenteritis, or other minor infections of the GI tract.

Safety: Sage leaf is safe, but it should be consumed only as a culinary herb during pregnancy. The essential oil is high in thujones, which can be toxic if taken in sufficient quantity, though there is little concern when used diluted in water as a mouth rinse or gargle and then spit out.

Skullcap herb (Scutellaria lateriflora)

Use: Skullcap is a member of the mint family native to eastern North America that has long been used as a relaxant and calmative. Early physicians prescribed it for mental or physical exhaustion, muscular spasms, tremors, and irritability and restlessness with nervous excitability and sleeplessness. Skullcap was listed in the *United States Pharmacopoeia* from 1860 until 1900, and in the *National Formulary* from 1916 to 1942. Scutellarin, a compound in skullcap, has mild sedative and antispasmodic properties.

Despite its widespread and strong historical use, there has been very little modern study of skullcap. Nineteen healthy volunteers were given a placebo capsule or 100-, 200-, or 350-milligram capsules of a freeze-dried extract of skullcap and asked to rate their anxiety an hour later. The volunteers taking the two higher doses of skullcap showed a reduction in anxiety levels.

Safety: Although cases of severe liver toxicity with skullcap have been reported, these were found to be due to the adulteration of skullcap products with a similar-appearing but dangerous plant, germander. Always purchase skullcap from a reputable manufacturer or supplier.

St. John's wort herb *(Hypericum perforatum)*

Use: St. John's wort is best known today for its use in the treatment of depression, although this herbal remedy has been used for at least two millennia for a variety of health conditions. Early physicians used it to treat mental and menstrual disorders, nerve pain, and stomach ulcers, and topically for the healing of wounds and burns.

Modern science is confirming what the ancients knew. In 2009, researchers evaluated 29 clinical trials conducted on St. John's wort for mild to moderate depression and concluded that it is more effective than placebo and is as effective as standard prescription antidepressants in terms of effectiveness with fewer adverse effects.

St. John's wort oil is also highly regarded as a topical agent. When the flowering tops are infused in oil, the oil turns a bright ruby red after sitting in the sun for several weeks. The oil is then massaged into the skin to relieve pain or made into an ointment and applied to skin to treat wounds, burns, and insect bites. Basic science and animal studies have now confirmed that the oil eases inflammation of the skin and also helps fight bacteria. St. John's wort is also highly effective against herpes simplex 1—the virus known to cause cold sores and fever blisters.

Safety: Although safe and effective, St. John's wort can interact with many medications. Always check with your health care provider or pharmacist before taking it internally if you're taking prescription medications.

Tea tree oil *(Melaleuca alternifolia)*

Use: Tea tree is a small tree native to the northeast coast of New South Wales, Australia. The leaves were used by the indigenous peoples for the treatment of fever, wounds, and as a refreshing tea. The first written medical testimony of tea tree was published in the *Medical Journal of Australia* in 1930, in which the use of tea tree oil was discussed as a wound disinfectant. The oil was issued as an antiseptic to soldiers during WWII. Over the past decades, the essential oil has been shown to be highly active against numerous pathogens including *Staphylococcus aureus, S. epidermidis, Propionibacterium acnes, Candida albicans,* and *Trichomonas vaginalis.* Studies have shown that tea tree oil applied topically can be effective against toenail fungus. A randomized clinical trial of 124 patients with acne found that a 5 percent tea tree oil gel was as effective as 5 percent benzoyl peroxide, but was better tolerated.

Safety: There are a number of case reports in the medical literature of dermatitis occurring after the topical application of tea tree oil. Except on toenails, always dilute the essential oil before applying. Tea tree oil is NOT safe for internal use.

Thyme herb *(Thymus vulgaris)*
Use: Thyme is one of our most revered herbs for the treatment of upper respiratory infection, cough, and congestion, and herbalists widely recognize its value as an adjunct therapy in asthma formulae. The German health authorities approve thyme for treating symptoms of bronchitis, whooping cough, and congestion of the upper respiratory tract.

Thyme's antitussive, expectorant, antimicrobial, and antispasmodic actions are attributed primarily to its flavonoids and the volatile oils thymol and carvacrol. Thymol is a potent antiseptic and one of the main ingredients in Listerine mouthwash. Thymol is also a potent antifungal agent, which is why the diluted tincture is used for infant thrush and vaginal yeast infections.

Safety: It is safe to use thyme as a seasoning during pregnancy, but medicinal doses of thyme should not be used during pregnancy.

Uva ursi leaves *(Arctostaphylos uva ursi)*

Use: Uva ursi, also known as bearberry, has long been used for the treatment of lower urinary tract infection and inflammation. The European Scientific Cooperative on Phytotherapy and British Herbal Medicine Association approve the use of uva ursi for inflammation/infection of the lower urinary tract. The leaves contain roughly 6 to 11 percent arbutin, the primary constituent responsible for its urinary antiseptic activity. Antibacterial testing shows that arbutin is highly active against *E. coli, Pseudomonas aeruginosa, Proteus mirabilis,* and *Staphylococcus aureus.* A double-blind, randomized study was conducted with 57 women who had experienced at least three bladder infections within the previous year that had been successfully treated with antibiotics. They received either uva ursi/dandelion or placebo tablets for a month. They were followed for a year, and any bladder infections were treated with antibiotics. None of the patients in the uva ursi group had a recurrence of bladder infection, compared to 23 percent of the placebo group.

Safety: Uva ursi is contraindicated during pregnancy and breast-feeding. Do not consume uva ursi for more than four weeks.

Valerian root *(Valeriana officinalis)*

Use: Valerian has been used to ease anxiety, nervousness, and insomnia for centuries. By the 18th century, it was a widely accepted sedative and was listed in the *National Formulary* as a sleep aid and anxiety treatment until 1950, when it was replaced by pharmaceutical sleeping agents. Valerian remains the most widely used sedative in Europe, where more than a hundred valerian preparations are sold in pharmacies across Germany, Belgium, France, Switzerland, and Italy. In human studies of valerian on its own, or in combination with hops, 12 of 16 found valerian improved sleep quality and shortened the time it takes to fall asleep. A clinical trial of valerian and lemon balm was shown to improve sleep in children 12 years of age and under. Valerian is a safe herbal choice for treating mild insomnia with the best studies suggesting it is more effective when used continuously for a period of two to four weeks, and the combination with hops and/or lemon balm may be more effective than valerian alone.

Safety: The *Botanical Safety Handbook* and the German health authorities do not list any contraindications for use in children or pregnancy. Because of its sedative effects, however, one should not drive or operate heavy machinery, or take in combination with other sedatives.

Witch hazel bark and leaves *(Hamamelis virginiana)*
Use: Witch hazel is indigenous to the United States and Canada and is widely used to relieve skin irritation, bruising, and hemorrhoids. Witch hazel leaf and bark have been valued for their astringent properties for centuries. The bark is generally much higher in tannins, the compounds that cause capillaries to constrict when applied topically to broken skin. This is one reason it works so well to reduce bleeding and swelling. It is found in a number of popular hemorrhoid creams, because witch hazel helps relieve itching and pain. It can be used to sooth poison ivy, poison oak, and chicken pox outbreaks.

Safety: There are no contraindications with topical application of witch hazel. Rare allergic reactions are possible.

Yarrow flowering tops *(Achillea millefolium)*
Use: Throughout Western history, there has probably not been a more famous wound healer than yarrow. Reportedly, Achilles received the gift of yarrow from Chiron, the wise centaur, who told the warrior to take it into battle with him to staunch the flow of blood in those who were wounded. From ancient Greece and Rome and throughout the Middle Ages, soldiers would rub

the flowering tops into injured tissue and wounds. Known as "soldier's woundwort," yarrow was carried by soldiers during the Civil War for the same purpose as their ancient counterparts.

The flowering tops are rich in tannins that act as astringents and achilletin and achilleine, constituents that stop the flow of blood. Camphor and eugenol provide mild analgesic properties, while azulene exerts anti-inflammatory activity. Yarrow may be safely used for open wounds with considerable swelling and edema.

Safety: Yarrow should not be used internally during pregnancy. Rare allergic reactions are possible.

Yerba santa leaves *(Eriodictyon californicum)*

Use: Yerba santa, or holy herb, is an indigenous evergreen aromatic shrub with a long history of use by the indigenous peoples living in what are now California, Arizona, and northern Mexico. The thick, sticky leaves were widely used to treat colds, asthma, bronchitis, and hay fever. It has a drying effect upon nasal and respiratory passages, making it wonderful for chronic congestion and for asthma with excessive bronchial secretions. The leaves are rich in phenols and resins that partially account for its expectorant and bronchial dilating effects. The phenols possess antiseptic and anti-inflammatory activity. Parke-Davis & Co. sold a pharmaceutical preparation of the plant that eventually became an official drug in the *United States Pharmacopoeia* from 1894 to 1905, and again from 1916 to 1947. Yerba santa is often partnered with grindelia in respiratory formulas, and like grindelia, it is highly effective for relieving the itch and redness of poison ivy or poison oak.

Safety: No safety concerns or contraindications are known; however, it is probably best to avoid in pregnancy.

Acknowledgments

This book was waiting for many years to be birthed. There are too many people to thank. I want to express my gratitude to Maggie Greenwood, Susan Hitchcock, and the team at National Geographic, who midwifed me through the process of writing this book. I could not have finished it without their patient guiding hands. I am so extremely grateful to my grandmothers for inspiring me to learn about the plants and healing. There are no words to express my gratitude to all the clients and patients who trusted me with their stories and allowed me to enter into their lives for a time. That bond is sacred to me. To all my brother and sister herbalists: Rosemary Gladstar, David Winston, Roy Upton, David Hoffman, Susun Weed, Aviva Romm, Tori Hudson, Mark Blumenthal, Deb Soule, Christopher Hobbs, and the late Michael Moore: Your wisdom and work continues to inspire me, as do the countless numbers of healers who have passed along their wisdom since antiquity.

To my beloved Jim, you are true north to me. Never wavering, always steady, so strong and tender. Thank you for encouraging me to write this book for our future generations. And to my wondrous children, Mekoce and Kiara, thank you for always being so patient on our endless herb-picking trips, helping on those nights we stayed up late making medicine, sharing your delight when you ate fresh peas or tomatoes from the garden, and believing in me all these years.

Finally, I would like to honor the plants themselves. While the plants could certainly live without us, we could not live without them. They are our very breath. They have been my green allies and elders for as long as I can remember. Teaching me how to grow and harvest them for food and medicine, showing me the places in the deserts and mountains they called home, and perhaps most of all, reminding me that being healthy is my birthright.

Index

STAY HEALTHY
with more books from National Geographic

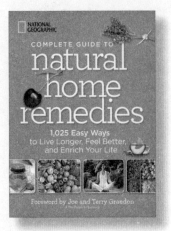

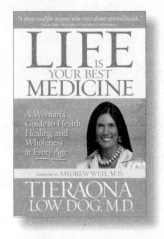

▲ This book features practical cures, medicinal herbs, healing foods, green housecleaning, sustainable cosmetics, alternative therapies, and tons of lifestyle changes tips.

▲ Dr. Low Dog weaves together the wisdom of traditional medicine and the knowledge of modern-day medicine into an elegant message of health and self-affirmation for women of every age.

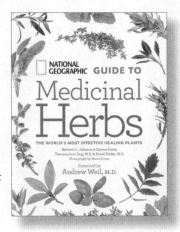

▶ Provides reliable and practical information about some of the most important medicinal herbs available.

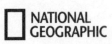

Like us on Facebook.com: Nat Geo Books

Follow us on Twitter.com: @NatGeoBooks

AVAILABLE WHEREVER BOOKS ARE SOLD
nationalgeographic.com/books